D1257794

The Vegetarian Cookbook

Publications International, Ltd.

Louis Weber, CEO
Publications International, Ltd.
7373 North Cicero Avenue
Lincolnwood, IL 60712

Pictured on the front cover *(clockwise from top left):* Chickpea Burger *(page 132),* French Carrot Quiche *(page 203)* and Quinoa and Mango Salad *(page 178).*

Pictured on the back cover *(left to right):* Seitan Fajitas *(page 292),* Barley and Vegetable Risotto *(page 135)* and Pear Gorgonzola Melts *(page 101).*

Photography on page 5 © Thinkstock
Photograph of cutting board on page 16 © PhotoSpin

Contributing writer: Marilyn Pocius

ISBN: 978-1-68022-144-2

Library of Congress Control Number: 2015938825

Manufactured in China.

8 7 6 5 4 3 2 1

Microwave Cooking: Microwave ovens vary in wattage. Use the cooking times as guidelines and check for doneness before adding more time.

Publications International, Ltd.

Contents

Introduction

What Does it Mean to Be Vegetarian?

Vegetarian, at least as defined for this book, means consuming no meat, poultry or fish. But there are many kinds of vegetarians and hundreds of reasons for being one. A recent study estimates that about 3.2 percent of adults in the U.S. (7.3 million people) follow a vegetarian-based diet; 15 million more say they follow a vegetarian-inclined diet. More people, especially young ones, are embracing a vegetarian lifestyle every day.

About half of the surveyed vegetarians said that the main reason they eat a plant-based diet is to improve overall health. A diet filled with veggies, fruits, grains and nuts tends to be lower in saturated fat than a meat-based diet and higher in fiber and antioxidants as well. We all know we should be eating more vegetables—it's the advice given by every nutritionist and on every food pyramid. Becoming vegetarian, even if it's only part time, is a great opportunity to do just that.

Sure there are health and environmental benefits to giving up meat, but one of the unsung joys of cooking vegetarian dishes is the incredible flavors you'll discover. There is so much variety in terms of color, taste and texture in the plant kingdom. When a meal isn't centered

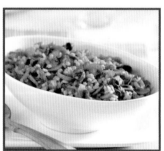

Barley and Vegetable Risotto, pg. 135

around meat, it's easier to appreciate the sweet tenderness of a roasted beet or the crunch of just-picked sugar snap peas. It's astonishing how delicious vegetables can be when prepared with recipes designed to make the most of them. Meat eaters don't know what they're missing when they dismiss vegetables as boring side dishes. There's nothing boring about Barley and Vegetable Risotto (page 135) or Butternut Gnocchi with Herb Butter (page 204)!

> ### Religion and Vegetarianism
>
> India has the world's largest population of vegetarians. This is no surprise since it is the birthplace of Hinduism, Jainism and Buddhism. All three of these religions favor vegetarianism as part of their nonviolent philosophy. Hare Krishnas, Seventh Day Adventists and Quakers also promote a plant-based diet.

The Many Flavors of Vegetarianism

Mainstream vegetarians are sometimes referred to as lacto-ovo vegetarians. (Lacto stands for milk; ovo for eggs.) They eat eggs, milk and dairy products in addition to plant-based foods. Lacto-vegetarians consume milk products, but not eggs. Pescatarians consume fish and other seafood, in addition to dairy and eggs. Vegans eat only plant-based foods—no dairy, eggs, cheese or honey. See page 8 for more information on the vegan diet.

Flexitarians are semi-vegetarians. They eat meat occasionally in small amounts, but derive the bulk of their calories from plants. This is a group that is growing in numbers rapidly as more people omit meat from their daily meals for health or environmental reasons.

Health is the most common reason for going vegetarian, but concern for animals is also part of the motivation. Many animal rights supporters simply feel that it is morally indefensible to kill animals for food. For others, the very idea of meat becomes repulsive once they accept reality—the shrink-wrapped pork chops in the meat case came from a cute pink pig, like Babe or Porky. In the age of instant information we can't ignore where our food comes from; the more we know about factory farms, mad-cow disease, E. coli contamination and the like, the more we lose our appetite for steak.

Vegetarian Goes Mainstream

Gone are the days when a vegetarian had to visit a strange smelling, brightly lit health food store to buy provisions. Now any decent size market stocks soymilk, quinoa, veggie burgers and even seitan. Certainly there are more vegetarians than ever, but there are also a lot of people who want the benefits of a vegetarian diet but don't want to commit to it 100 percent. As they discover how delicious vegetarian cuisine can be, they want to have their tofu and eat

Diet for a Small Planet

American vegetarianism really caught on in 1971 with the publication of a runaway bestseller by Frances Moore Lappé—*Diet for a Small Planet.* The book encouraged people to give up meat because it wasted resources that could be used to feed a hungry world. It inspired millions. Vegetarian cookbooks, restaurants, co-ops and communes became commonplace.

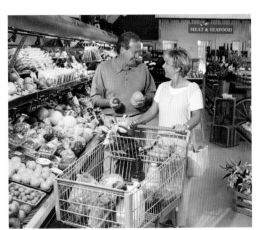

chicken, too. Some people simply give up beef and pork (these folks are sometimes labeled "pollotarians"). Others are vegetarian most of the time but break the rules for special occasions or when a serious craving hits.

Whether they're called flexitarians or semi-vegetarians, these advocates of eating less meat are a huge segment of the population. Often they transition to becoming true vegetarians. Almost always they realize that vegetarian cuisine can open up whole new worlds of flavor and enjoyment.

Planning Vegetarian Meals

For some time now, American meals have consisted of a main course—meat—accompanied by sides. The newly minted vegetarian may, at first, simply replace the center-of-the-plate meat with a veggie lasagna or tofu dog. A meal certainly doesn't have to be structured that way. It doesn't even have to be served on one big plate! In fact, most cuisines around the world are considerably less meat-centric. In Chinese and Japanese cooking, meat is more often considered a condiment or flavoring agent than the star of the show. The Middle East has its small plates called mezes and Spain specializes in tapas.

Vegetarian meals work well as a series of individual dishes that complement each other without a single item stealing the show. Soup, salad and a crusty loaf of bread can be a filling and delightful dinner. A vegetable gratin, a colorful stir-fry or a cheese soufflé could be the centerpiece for an elegant dinner party. The possibilities are endless.

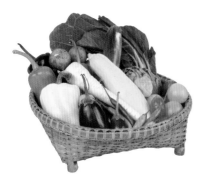

Color it Delicious

There are more colorful options to choose with veggies, fruits and grains than you would ever find with meat. Variety is an important ingredient in any meal, especially a vegetarian one. Choosing a colorful array of foods doesn't just look pretty, it provides a good range of vitamins, minerals and micronutrients. The colors can come in a series of smaller dishes—a green salad, cornbread, black beans and rice—or you can mix colorful vegetables in an Asian-style stir-fry or other main course.

Think Different

Think out of the box when it comes to traditional dishes. A salad doesn't have to be the standard lettuce with dressing. It can also be an exotic Mixed Grain Tabbouleh (page 164), sliced tomatoes with avocado or just an assortment of crisp raw veggies. Turn a favorite vegetable into a casserole or gratin to make it more filling. Resize an appetizer recipe and call it a main course (or vice versa). If you've got a taste for a popular meat-containing dish like lasagna or fajitas, indulge in it vegetarian style. Try Pesto Lasagna (page 258) or Seitan Fajitas (page 292).

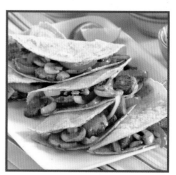

Seitan Fajitas
pg. 292

The Vegetarian Pantry

All cooking depends on the quality of ingredients—even more so if it's vegetarian. The sometimes subtle flavors of fresh produce need to be coaxed and complemented, not overwhelmed. Use cheap oil or a dusty jar of dried basil and it will be easy to tell. The flavor of meat can mask a multitude of sins!

For the recipes in this book, here are some pantry items you should keep on hand:

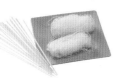 Asian noodles:
rice noodles, soba

 Bulgur wheat

 Cornmeal

 Lentils

 Pasta

 Rice:
long grain,
brown, basmati,
jasmine

 Tomatoes:
canned whole
and diced

 Beans:
a variety of
canned or dried

 Chickpeas

 Dried mushrooms

 Oils:
extra virgin olive
oilvegetable oil

 Quinoa

 Soy sauce

 Vegetable broth

Vegan Cooking

In addition to eliminating meat, fish and poultry from their diets, vegans also cut out other animal products, including dairy, eggs and honey. Dairy products are usually the most difficult to replace. For most recipes, soymilk or other dairy-free milk can be substituted one for one. Butter can often be replaced with dairy-free margarine, but read labels carefully since many margarines contain milk products in the form of casein or whey. There are vegan forms of mayonnaise readily available.

Cheese is trickier. It can usually be left out entirely if it's only a topping or minor part of the recipe. Cheese alternatives are available but don't always taste or melt like cheese and texture can be a problem if they are an important element in the recipe. For gratins or casseroles, try a bread crumb or nut topping in place of cheese. Crumbled tofu is also a possibility.

Commercial vegan egg replacements are available. (Don't be fooled by the cholesterol-free egg substitutes in the dairy case; they're egg whites.) Many recipes, including soufflés and fritattas, can't be recreated without eggs. For others, especially baked goods than use no more than 3 eggs, fruit purées or silken tofu are good substitutes. Use ¼ cup of tofu, ¼ cup of applesauce or one mashed banana to fill in for one egg.

Vitamins and Minerals

Every diet needs variety to be healthy. A vegetarian diet consisting of macaroni and cheese and pizza would certainly not provide the vitamins, minerals and other nutrients human bodies need. A diet of fast food burgers, fried chicken and soda would be even worse! See the chart on page 11 for some sources of nutrients most often derived from animal products that are of particular concern to vegetarians. Vegans have to be even more aware. Vitamin B-12 especially can be hard to obtain for those who omit dairy and eggs.

The key to healthy eating is the same for vegetarians, vegans, flexitarians and meat eaters: enjoy a wide variety of food every day.

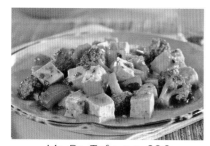

Ma Po Tofu, pg. 290

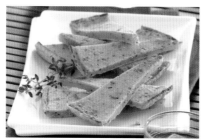

Socca, pg. 46

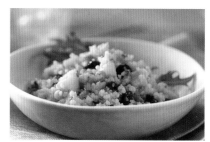

Quinoa and Mango Salad, pg. 178

What about Wine?

Enjoying a glass of wine with dinner is certainly a pleasure that shouldn't be denied vegetarians. The rules for pairing are in the same spirit as for a meat-based meal, but instead of red with meat, white with poultry and fish, serve heavier red wines with hearty, starchy dishes and whites with lighter green vegetable dishes. As always, your own preferences are the only important deciding factor.

These wines pair well with...	these dishes
crisp clean whites (Sauvingon Blanc, Champagne, Pino Grigio)	veggie risottos, quiches, pasta primavera
full-bodied whites (Chardonnay, Viognier)	creamy, rich dishes, fettucine Alfredo
fruity reds (Beaujoulais, Merlot, Rioja)	bean and cheese dishes, mushroom dishes
hearty reds (Chianti, Cabernet, Zinfandel)	lasagna, root vegetables, chillies and hearty soups, lentils

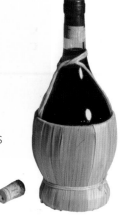

Keep Things Interesting

1. Serve three or four small plates instead of one main course plus sides.

2. Go ethnic. Explore vegetarian Italian pastas and risotto, Asian stir-fries, Mexican bean dishes or French soufflés.

3. Serve breakfast for dinner. Eggs, waffles and pancakes taste great late.

4. Give potatoes and pasta a rest. Try adding couscous, quinoa, barley, bulgur wheat and brown rice to your repertoire.

5. Experiment with meat replacements, including tofu, seitan and tempeh.

6. Cook with the seasons. Take advantage of farmers' markets and enjoy fresh produce every day.

The Healthy Vegetarian Diet

Vegetarianism has come a long way from the dark days when it was considered a sort of fringe behavior that often involved living in a commune. Even fast food spots now offer vegetarian options. In fact, the American Dietetic Association, a fairly conservative organization, recently issued a position paper that said appropriately planned vegetarian diets are "healthful, nutritionally adequate, and may provide health benefits in the prevention and treatment of certain diseases." The paper added that being vegetarian was appropriate for just about anyone, including children, adolescents, pregnant women and athletes.

The Protein Problem that Isn't

Some of the old myths never die, and if you've been a vegetarian for any length of time you've probably been asked, "But what do you do about protein?" Our meat-centric society generally thinks of beef, pork and chicken as the only "good" sources of protein.

Protein is part of the structure of every cell in our bodies. When protein from food is digested it is broken down into amino acids. These in turn are reassembled into the proteins our body uses. Decades ago it was believed that since meat contained all the essential amino acids (see the sidebar for a definition), vegetarians needed to eat a combination of foods at each meal that provided this same assortment. *Diet for a Small Planet* and other books of the time called this "protein combining." It was complicated and soon found to be unnecessary.

What's an essential amino acid?

The human body can produce the amino acids it requires to make protein, except for eight of them. These are called the essential amino acids and must be obtained from food. Animal products contain all eight. Most plant sources lack some of them. The exceptions are soybeans and quinoa, which, like meat, are complete proteins.

While plant sources don't contain all 10 amino acids, they do contain an assortment. As long as you eat a variety of food every day and get enough calories, your metabolism will take care of the combining for you. There's no reason for vegetarians who are eating a wholesome diet to worry about protein intake. In fact, next time someone asks you about it, you might point out that most Americans get too much protein, which can definitely be unhealthy.

Know Your Nutrients

Here's a list of good sources of nutrients sometimes missing from a vegetarian diet.

Protein	Vitamin B-12	Zinc
dairy products	dairy products	legumes
eggs	eggs	nuts
legumes	enriched soymilk	soy products
lentils	fortified cereals	sprouts
soy products	nutritional yeast	whole grains
whole grains		wheat germ

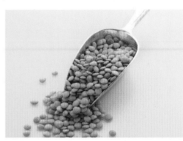

Calcium	Iron*
broccoli	beans, peas and lentils
dairy products	dried fruit
enriched soymilk	enriched cereals
kale	kale
spinach	spinach
	whole grains

*To enhance iron absorption, combine these foods with those rich in Vitamin C.

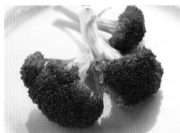

What's Nutritional Yeast?

It's not for making bread rise! Nutritional yeast is a favorite with vegetarians, especially vegans, since it has a taste similar to Parmesan cheese and can be a source of vitamin B-12. It comes in powder or flake form and can be sprinkled directly on food or used in recipes. Read labels carefully though, since only a few brands are fortified with B-12. The tongue twister of the chemical name for B-12 you should look for is cyanocobalamin.

Vegetable Basics

Fresh vs. Frozen vs. Canned

Say yes to all three! Fresh produce picked at the peak of ripeness is certainly the tastiest and most nutritious choice. Too bad we don't all have year-round vegetable gardens in our backyards. In the real world there are plenty of times when fresh just isn't an option. Frozen vegetables are usually picked at peak ripeness and blanched before flash freezing so they retain most of their vitamins and minerals. In fact, frozen can be better for you than out of season produce that's traveled cross-country losing nutrients all the way. Canned products are convenient and belong in every pantry. Without canned tomatoes and beans, being a vegetarian would be a lot tougher. The most important thing is to eat more vegetables and fruits and a greater variety of them.

Give Me Some Skin

Drop that peeler! The skin is often the most nutritious part of a vegetable. There's really no need to eliminate the peel on a potato, a summer squash or even a carrot unless it's really thick or the vegetable is bruised. Just scrub well and enjoy.

Shopping for Fresh Produce

Most of us shop for family meals in a supermarket and we're always looking for the best prices. Produce departments offer a huge selection of veggies and fruits and the good news is that often the biggest bargain is also the best choice. What's on sale is usually what's in season and that's tops for nutrition and taste. Flavor and texture vary depending on the freshness of the vegetable, how it was handled, what variety it is, how it was grown and even the soil it was grown in. Often commercial growers pick the varieties that are easiest to ship, last the longest or look prettiest. This does not always result in the best taste. Don't just choose the biggest, shiniest item in the bin. Feel it for firmness and rely on your sense of smell, too. A simple sniff of a melon or tomato can reveal a great deal.

The growth of farmers' markets has made vegetarian shopping a lot more fun. Make time to explore a market near you. Farmers and fellow shoppers will often be happy to share preparation tips and recipes. Ethnic markets are another great source for produce. Frequently stores that cater to Latin American, Italian, Asian or other clientele offer a wider selection and better prices. You'll be surprised at how many delicious kinds of eggplant there are that don't show up in an ordinary supermarket.

Keeping It Fresh

Most, but not all, fresh produce lasts longer if stored in the refrigerator. The vegetable crisper drawer is designed is to keep in humidity and protect veggies from the drier refrigerator air. Newer fridges often have a sliding tab on the front of the drawers that allows you to make further adjustments. Fruits usually require less humidity than vegetables.

Some fruits produce ethylene gas as they ripen. These include apples, avocados, bananas, peaches, plums, melons and tomatoes. Some vegetables are sensitive to ethylene and will spoil more quickly if exposed to it. Lettuce gets brown spots and broccoli buds may turn yellow. Be careful to keep the ethylene-producing fruits separate from broccoli, leafy greens, beans, carrots, cucumbers, eggplant, peas and peppers.

COOL Labeling

As of 2008, retailers are required by law to indicate what country the produce they sell came from. The law is called COOL, which stands for Country Of Origin Labeling. So now you can choose to buy apples from the U.S. or avoid garlic from China. Pretty cool, isn't it?

For maximum storage time, it's best to store produce unwashed. On the other hand, if you know you won't find the time during a busy workweek, fill the sink with water and take care of a big load all at once. Prepping vegetables ahead sometimes also makes sense. They won't keep as long, but you may be more likely to enjoy a pasta and veggie dinner if you can get it on the table faster. If you do prep before refrigerating, drain the produce well and store it in a plastic bag, preferably perforated. Add some paper towels to absorb any excess moisture. See the chart on the next page for more storage and freshness information.

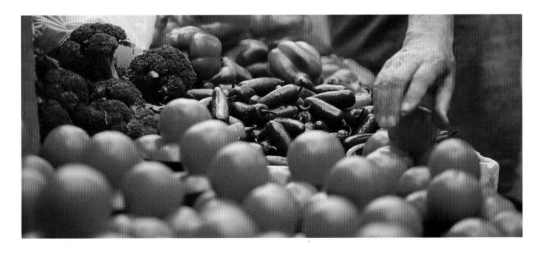

Introduction

VEGETABLE	HOW TO STORE	USE WITHIN...
Artichokes	refrigerate, wrapped	7 days
Asparagus	refrigerate, wrap stalks in damp towel or place in glass with water	3 to 4 days
Beans, green snap, wax	refrigerate, unwashed in plastic bag	3 to 5 days
Beets	refrigerate, unwashed in plastic bag	2 weeks
Bell peppers, whole	refrigerate in crisper in plastic bag	1 to 2 weeks
Broccoli	refrigerate, unwashed in plastic bag	3 to 5 days
Cabbage	refrigerate, unwashed in plastic bag	1 to 2 weeks
Carrots, unpeeled	remove tops; refrigerate in plastic bag	3 to 4 weeks
Carrots, peeled and/or cut up, "baby" carrots	refrigerate, wrapped tightly in covered container	2 to 3 weeks
Celery	refrigerate in plastic bag or covered container	1 to 2 weeks
Chili peppers	refrigerate in crisper in plastic bag	1 week
Corn on the cob	refrigerate, unhusked and uncovered	1 to 2 days
Cucumber	refrigerate, unwashed in plastic bag	1 week
Eggplant	refrigerate, unwashed, in plastic bag	5 to 7 days
Garlic, whole bulb	store, uncovered at cool room temperature	3 to 5 months
Greens, salad	refrigerate, unwashed, in plastic bag	up to 1 week
Greens: kale, collards	refrigerate, unwashed, in plastic bag	5 days
Mushrooms, whole	refrigerate, unwashed, in *paper* bag	4 to 5 days
Mushrooms, sliced	refrigerate in covered container	1 to 2 days
Onions, whole	store in cool (50–60°F), dark place or refrigerate; do not store near potatoes*	2 to 3 months
Peas	refrigerate, unshelled, in plastic bag	3 to 5 days
Potatoes	store in cool (50–60°F), dark place; do not store near onions*	2 to 3 months
Spinach	refrigerate, unwashed, in plastic bag	3 to 5 days
Squash, summer	refrigerate, unwashed in plastic bag	4 to 5 days
Squash, winter	store in cool (50–60°F), dry place	1 to 2 months
Sweet potatoes	store in cool (50–60°F), dark place	1 month
Tomatoes	store at room temperature	1 to 5 days

*Never store potatoes near onions. It speeds spoilage of both due to a chemical reaction between them.

The Well-Equipped Vegetarian

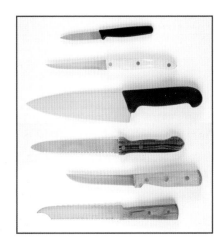

Knife Know-How

It's not that vegetarian cooking is different, but there are certain tools that can make it more enjoyable. (With what you're saving on groceries, you're entitled to treat yourself!) A sharp knife is the foundation of every good cook's kitchen kit. It makes chopping and slicing easier and neater and it's also safer. A dull knife is more likely to slip. Sharp knives slide through vegetables without crushing them and this can actually improve flavor and texture, too. If you've ever pulsed an onion for a bit too long in a food processor only to have it turn to watery mush, you get the idea.

Choosing the right knife has been the subject of many articles and you can easily do some research to understand the details we don't have room to handle here. The simplest rule, and one that is often overlooked, is that it's important to hold a knife to see how it fits in your hand and get a feel for weight and balance. A good knife should be an extension of the cook's hand.

It's just as important to keep your knives sharp as it is to buy good ones. Many hardware and cooking supply stores will sharpen your knives for a small fee. You can also buy an electric or manual sharpener to use at home. The steel (a metal rod mounted on a handle) is used to maintain the edge of your knives, but cannot actually sharpen them once they become dull. There's no need to have dozens of different knives. A good chef's knife, paring knife and a serrated knife (for tomatoes and bread) can handle just about any job.

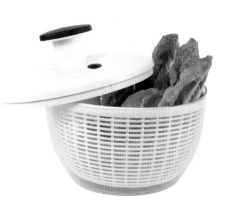

A Washday Miracle!

One of the most time-consuming chores for the vegetarian cook is washing vegetables and the peskiest things to clean are greens like spinach and lettuce. Grit can hide in the leaves unless they are thoroughly swished underwater. Invest in a salad spinner if you haven't already. They come in a variety of styles, including those with a push-button or pull-string for spinning. Fill the sink with water, put the greens in the basket and swish away. Lift the basket out of the sink and spin dry, leaving dirt and grit behind.

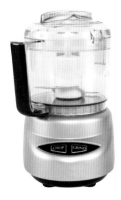

Power on Tap

The vegetarian kitchen makes good use of food processors and blenders. They make shredding cabbage for a salad, puréeing a soup or preparing pesto a breeze. In addition to a full-size processor, a mini with only a one- or two-cup capacity can be handy for small amounts of veggies, herbs or nuts. A blender is a must if you make smoothies, and it can also make creamy dips, soups and sauces. An immersion blender (the kind that you stick into the pot) is not as powerful but can be useful if you make a lot of soups; you won't have to transfer hot liquid to and from a regular blender or processor.

Pots, Pans, Skillets, Etc.

A big (2-gallon) stockpot will serve you well for making soup, blanching vegetables and cooking pasta. You'll also need a large ovenproof Dutch oven or deep skillet with a lid for making stews and braising. A small and/or medium saucepan can take care of steaming or boiling. You'll need small and medium skillets for sautéing as well as a large (12-inch) deep skillet for preparing stir-fries, one-dish meals and large quantities of vegetables.

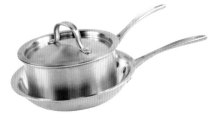

For use in the oven, a large metal roasting pan and a rimmed baking sheet (sometimes called a jelly-roll pan) are the minimum. You probably already have an assortment of smaller baking dishes and casseroles. It's nice to have a gratin dish and a soufflé dish as well, though a casserole can usually fill in.

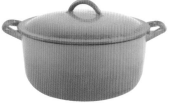

A large cutting board is essential—at least 10×12 inches. Smaller boards are frustrating. They don't give you room to safely chop an entire bunch of parsley or an eggplant without things falling off the edges. It's best to have more than one cutting board so you don't have to keep washing and drying between tasks. Plastic has the advantage of usually being dishwasher safe, but wood boards are also a fine choice. If the board slides around while you're working, anchor it by placing a damp towel underneath.

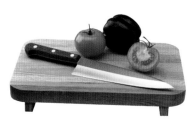

If you enjoy grilling, it's worth investing in a vegetable grill basket or grill-topper. These useful tools allow you to grill small items or small pieces of larger ones without anything falling through the grate. A perforated metal steamer that fits inside a saucepan or an Asian bamboo steamer can also come in handy.

Beyond Broccoli

Most folks who say they can't imagine what vegetarians eat lack imagination themselves! The plant kingdom offers choices of color, texture and taste that go way beyond the dull beige world of meat. Nevertheless, it is easy to get stuck in a rut and keep repeating the same old broccoli, corn and zucchini. Here are some ideas for moving beyond the usual veggie rotation.

Artichokes

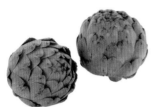

Fresh artichokes' peak season is the early spring. In additionto the familiar globe artichoke, you will sometimes see fresh baby artichokes. They usually don't have a choke that has to be removed and they are tender enough to cook quickly. Frozen and canned artichoke hearts are excellent items to have on hand. Jarred marinated hearts are packed in oil and add a different flavor to dishes.

Bok choy and other Asian greens

In Chinese the word "choy" means greens. Bok choy with crisp white stalks and dark green leaves is the most common. What is sometimes labeled baby bok choy is a miniature jade green variety. There is also choy sum (white flowering cabbage). They all have a mild cabbage flavor and can be used interchangeably with each other and in other cabbage recipes, so don't hesitate to try something new.

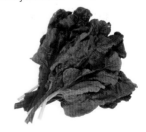

Chayote and other summer squash

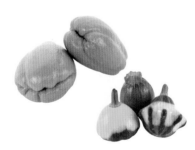

There are dozens of kinds of summer squash besides zucchini. Chayote, which is sometimes called mirliton, is light green and pear-shaped. The flavor is mild and a bit sweet. Even the stone in the center is edible (and delicious). There are also pattypan squash, which look like cute flying saucers, and a round zucchini-like squash sometimes labeled "8 ball squash." All of these can be used interchangeably although cooking times will need to be adjusted.

Chard

Sometimes called *Swiss chard*, this gorgeous "green" comes in a rainbow of hues. Stems can be thick or thin, red, yellow or white. It is related to beets and spinach and tastes a bit like both. Stems take longer to cook than the leaves, so give them a head start.

Introduction

Eggplant

If you are only familiar with the big purple globe eggplant available year round, you're in for a treat. Check a farmers' market or ethnic produce department in the summer and you'll find a huge variety. Slender Asian eggplants are shades of purple or striped with white. There are egg-size white eggplants—yes, that's where the name came from—and even reddish-orange and pale green varieties. In season, eggplant should have firm flesh with very little in the way of developed seeds. There's no need to peel or salt most varieties since they won't have the bitterness that puts some people off.

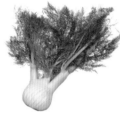

Fennel

Crisp, juicy fennel is an Italian vegetable that is finally being appreciated here. You will also see fennel labeled "finocchio" or "anise." Fennel can be enjoyed raw and sliced thin in a salad. Cooked, fennel's flavor mellows and sweetens. Add fennel to pasta dishes and mixed roasted vegetables.

Leeks

They look like green onions on steroids, but leeks, although related to onions, can play a different leading role. Once cooked, leeks soften and add sweet complexity to soups, stews, casseroles and other dishes. It is crucial to clean leeks thoroughly since mud hides deep between the leaves. Make sure to slit the leek horizontally and swish under copious amounts of water until the water runs clear.

Mushrooms

Pity the poor white button mushroom, which has now been upstaged by so many other tasty varieties. The brown *cremini* is actually the same type of mushroom as the white, just a different strain. And a *cremini* left to mature to its full adult size is the much-loved *portobello*. Shiitake mushrooms are now available fresh. The dried *shiitake*, also called Chinese black mushroom, is most likely familiar to anyone who has dined in a Chinese restaurant. Fresh *shiitakes* offer a milder version of the rich, meaty flavor of dried. Seek out those with thick, firm caps and a fresh aroma. *Oyster mushrooms* grow in thick clusters with overlapping leaflike caps. Their flavor is mild and their texture slightly chewy. You will often find a mix of the mushrooms just described packaged together and labeled "wild mushrooms." They are, almost always, not truly wild, but cultivated versions of what exists in the wild.

Root vegetables

Root veggies won't win any beauty contests, but what they lack in looks they more than make up in flavor. Roasted or braised, they turn soft and seductive. The two most popular roots—carrots and potatoes—are regulars in most kitchens, but there are many delicious options to explore.

Celery root may be the ugliest of the bunch. This large gnarly bulb, which is also called celeriac or knob celery, has a tough exterior covered in deep furrows. Don't try to peel celery root with an ordinary peeler; remove its outer shell with a paring knife. It can be used in gratins, mashed with potatoes, roasted or even used raw for a famous French café slaw: celeri remoulade. The flavor is like celery, only deeper.

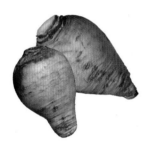

Rutabagas look like bigger, brawnier turnips and are related. Their exteriors are dark yellow with a purple blush and are often heavily waxed to keep them fresh. Inside, a rutabaga's flesh is a pale yellow. Like turnips, rutabagas are tastiest when young and not too big. *Kohlrabi* is actually a member of the cabbage family. The golf to tennis ball-size bulbs are pale green or purple outside. The flesh is crisp and has a broccoli-like flavor. Enjoy kohlrabi raw, or prepare it steamed, sauteed or roasted to bring out its sweetness.

If it looks like a carrot only white, it's probably a *parsnip*. These delicious roots may be the most under appreciated of all. Steamed, braised, roasted or pureed, parsnips are low in calories and high in fiber and have a light, earthy sweetness. Their flavor is even sweeter when they're harvested after a frost.

Winter squash

From the large *butternut* to the diminutive *delicata*, winter squash come in a boggling array of sizes and colors. Aside from Halloween pumpkins (good for toasted seeds and jack-o'-lanterns, but not for cooking), the largest variety that is readily available and offers good flavor is the smooth, beige *butternut squash*. This slightly sweet, rich tasting squash is classic in almost any preparation from soup to risotto. *Delicata squash* has recently become available and can be used like the more common acorn. This green-striped oblong squash cooks up tender with a buttery texture and a flavor reminiscent of corn. *Spaghetti squash* is like no other. It looks like a rounded golden football and when cooked yields crisp-tender strands that look like, and can be sauced like, you guessed it, spaghetti!

Going with the Grain

Grains are the center of the plate in many cultures. Asian cuisine is built around rice. In Thailand the traditional greeting translates as, "Have you eaten rice yet?" Italy has pasta made from durum wheat. In both North and South America, corn was central to ancient cuisine and culture. Bread and cereal are certainly mainstays of our lives, but fortunately there are more kinds of grains now available than ever and there are delicious options that go way beyond a loaf of white bread.

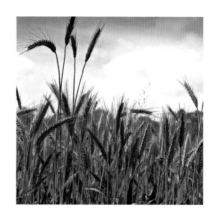

Storing Grains

Whole grains are considerably more nutritious than processed ones, but since they contain the oil-rich germ as well as the bran, they become rancid much more quickly. It's best to store what you won't use up in several months in the refrigerator or freezer. Buy small quantities of an assortment of grains and keep them in covered containers labeled with the date they were purchased. If you are buying from bulk bins, take a good sniff first. Grain should smell sweet and earthy not stale or rancid. Grains that are past their prime not only don't taste good, they take longer to cook.

barley

Slightly sweet, nutty and chewy, barley is easy to love and makes a good substitute for rice. Pearl (pearled) barley, which is the most available kind, has been polished to remove its tough outer hull. Hulled or Scotch barley has more of the bran intact so is more nutritious but also takes longer to cook.

bulgur wheat

To make bulgur wheat, whole kernels are steamed, dried and ground to varying degrees. The fine grind, which is the most common type, is ready in a matter of minutes. Bulgur is traditionally served cold in tabbouleh salad, but its fluffy texture also makes it a natural for soaking up juices or broths.

The Kernel of the Matter

All grains have three parts. There is a tough outer layer that protects the grain called the bran. The starchy endosperm makes up the biggest portion of the kernel. The germ or the embryo of the grain is at its base. The bran and the germ contain the most fiber and nutrients; they are the parts often removed when grain is processed. Whole grains still contain all three parts.

---

cornmeal/polenta

Polenta is the Italian name for a creamy porridge made from cornmeal that is eaten hot or cooled, sliced and fried. The American version of this dish would be called cornmeal mush. It's easy to see why it never caught on under that name! Polenta is most nutritious and flavorful if prepared from whole grain, stone-ground cornmeal.

couscous

We call couscous a grain, but it's actually a form of tiny pasta made from wheat flour. Whole wheat couscous is just as convenient as regular since it cooks in the same amount of time.

millet

Mild-mannered millet has small beadlike grains that cook quickly. Once considered "for the birds", millet is being recognized for its pleasant cornlike flavor and good nutritional profile—millet is rich in B vitamins.

> ### Grains as Convenience Foods
>
> It's true that whole grains take time to cook, but there's an easy way to enjoy them even on a busy weeknight. Stockpile! Instead of preparing just 1 cup of rice, barley, quinoa or whatever, double or triple the recipe and store the rest. Cooked grains will keep for several days in the refrigerator and for months in the freezer.

quinoa

If you're only going to add one new grain to your meals, make it quinoa. The Incas considered it sacred and called it the mother of all grains. Quinoa has also been called a supergrain since it is rich in protein, contains all essential amino acids, and is a good source of fiber, magnesium and iron. Oh, yes, it is also easy to digest, has a sweet subtle taste and cooks in about 15 minutes!

rice

Brown rice is whole grain rice with the nutrients in the bran or germ intact. There are many varieties of rice and they are often categorized by the length of their grains. *Long-grain rice* is at least three times longer than it is wide. These rices include the aromatic *jasmine* and *basmati* rices. *Short-grain rice* has plumper, rounder grains that tend to stick together more when cooked. Sushi rice and arborio rice are two examples. Rice that is especially sticky is often used in Asian desserts and is sometimes labeled *sweet or glutinous rice*, despite the fact that it contains no gluten!

wheat berries

These kernels of wheat are sold under the name whole wheat or wheat berries. The color of the berries (which are actually kernels) varies from reddish brown to pale cream. Wheat berries have a hearty, nutty flavor and satisfying chewiness. They can take up to an hour to cook, but the time can be shortened by presoaking.

The Beauty of Beans

Beans are one of the least expensive forms of protein. They are high in fiber and low in fat and come in a kaleidoscope of colors and shapes. Beans can be enjoyed in every kind of dish from a dip or a salad to stews and soups to hearty main courses. In Asia, sweetened red beans are dessert—they are used to fill pastries and even make ice cream!

adzuki beans
These small, dark red beans are slightly sweet and creamy when cooked. They are the basis for sweet red bean paste used in Asian desserts.

black beans (turtle beans, frijoles negros)
Black beans are a staple of Latin American dishes. Their strong, earthy flavor and firm texture help them stand out in soups, salads and all sorts of side dishes.

cannellini beans (white kidney beans)
Mild-tasting meaty cannellinis are often used in minestrone soup and other Italian dishes.

chickpeas (garbanzo beans)
The versatile chickpea has an almost buttery flavor and is a nutritional powerhouse with over 80 nutrients, plus plenty of fiber and protein. Many classic vegetarian dishes, including hummus and falafel, are based on the versatile chickpea.

kidney beans
Kidney beans are full-flavored and retain their kidney shape even with long cooking times. They are usually the bean of choice for chili or cold salads. They come in dark red, light red, pink or white (see cannellini beans).

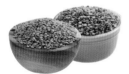

lentils
Lentils cook quickly and are often served puréed. The most common varieties are brown and red, but for a larger selection explore the many different kinds used in Indian or Middle Eastern cuisines.

lima beans (butter beans)
Pale green limas are starchy and satisfying. Their rich buttery flavor holds up better when they're fresh or frozen.

pinto beans
Speckled beige beans with darker streaks, pintos are used for refried beans, chili and many Mexican recipes. Unfortunately their pretty markings—"pinto" means painted in Spanish—turn a dull pinkish beige after cooking.

white beans (Great Northern, navy beans)
These mild, meaty beans are favorites in casseroles, stews and soups.

What's the difference between a bean and a legume?

Legumes are a class of vegetable that includes beans, peas and lentils, all of which grow in pods. What about green beans? When the entire pod is eaten, the plant is considered a green vegetable.

Dry Bean Basics

Cooking dried beans is easy, economical and produces firmer, tastier beans. It does take more time than opening a can, but most of it is unsupervised.

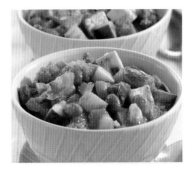

1. Buy the right beans. Old beans or those that have been stored in heat or humidity will never cook correctly. (Throw away that old package that's been in your cupboard for five years right now!) Purchase beans from a place that has a big turnover. Choose beans that are brightly colored with smooth skins.

Zesty Vegetarian Chili, pg. 98

2. Soak. Sort through the beans and discard any broken ones or foreign matter while rinsing them thoroughly. Place in a nonreactive bowl or pan and cover with fresh cold water by about 3 inches. Toss any beans that float. Soak at least four hours or overnight until the bean skins get wrinkled. (There is no need to soak lentils.)

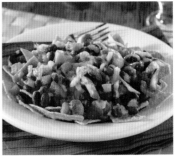

3. Cook. Drain the beans and rinse them. Place them in a saucepan and cover with at least one inch of water. Bring the beans to a boil and skim any foam that rises to the top. Cover and simmer the beans over low heat for 45 minutes to 2 hours or until tender but not mushy. Timing will

Black Bean and Mushroom Chilaquiles, pg. 152

depend on the variety of bean and also how long it was stored. Add hot water if needed to keep the beans covered. Add salt and seasonings when the beans are almost tender.

Bean Counting

One pound of dried beans will yield four to five cups of cooked beans, or approximately 8 servings. A 15-ounce can contains between 1½ to 2 cups of cooked beans, depending on the variety.

Using Your Noodles

Pasta may be a vegetarian's best friend! It's economical, versatile and easy to prepare. You can stuff it, sauce it, stir-fry it, bake it or make it into a fried cake. You can buy it dried in a box, fresh and in more shapes and colors than we have room for here. Besides Italian pasta, there are dozens of kinds of Asian noodles. Some are practically identical to their Italian counterparts, while others are made of different ingredients and require different cooking methods.

Does shape matter?

That depends on the recipe and your personal preferences. Obviously you wouldn't try to make lasagna with elbow macaroni. Although if you layered the cooked elbows with sauce and cheese, you'd end up with something delicious— it just wouldn't be called lasagna! Common sense and tradition indicate that a chunky sauce works better if there's a shape to catch it, like shells or orecchiette. For a soup, you need a shape that fits into a spoon. And for stuffing you need a shape that's big enough to fit a spoon in!

Umami: The Fifth Flavor

In addition to sweet, sour, salty and bitter, there is a taste that can be described as savoriness or meatiness. Called "umami" from the Japanese, this taste is present in meat, but also in mushrooms, soy sauce and other fermented soy products, cheese, ripe tomatoes, wine and balsamic vinegar. To add full-bodied savor to vegetarian dishes, add umami ingredients.

ASIAN NOODLES

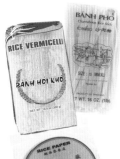
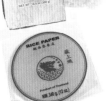

Soba noodles are flat Japanese noodles made with buckwheat flour, which gives them an earthy, nutty flavor. They are served cold during hot Japanese summers and hot in winter soups. Soba should be cooked until tender, not al dente.

Rice noodles come in a dizzying array of sizes and go by a number of names—rice sticks and rice vermicelli are two. Unlike soba or pasta, rice noodles only need to be soaked in hot water before using.

Chinese wheat noodles (mein) are similar to pasta and come in just as many styles and shapes with or without the addition of egg. They are cooked like pasta, too, and you can substitute a similar pasta shape if you have trouble finding the real thing.

Rice papers are translucent round sheets made from rice flour and water. They need only to be soaked for 20 seconds before being used to wrap ingredients.

The Pasta Cooking Quiz

There is a lot written about the simple art of cooking pasta, some of it contradictory. Test your knowledge with this quiz.

1. **What's the best way to cook pasta?**

a. Place it in several quarts of cold water and bring to a boil.

b. Add pasta to boiling water, add salt and cover the pot.

c. Bring an abundant quantity of salted water to a boil. Add pasta, stir and boil uncovered.

2. **How much salt should you add to pasta water?**

a. None. Pasta should be salted after cooking.

b. Two teaspoons

c. Enough to make it taste like the sea.

3. **You should add a tablespoon of olive oil to pasta cooking water...**

a. if you're worried about the pasta sticking together.

b. if you will be using a low-fat sauce.

c. Never!

4. **How do you tell when pasta is done?**

a. You follow the directions on the box and add a few minutes.

b. You throw it against the wall and see if it sticks.

c. You taste it.

5. **What does al dente mean?**

a. Pasta shaped like little teeth.

b. It's a small town in the Italian hills known for great pasta.

c. Literally "to the tooth." It's a description of perfectly cooked pasta that retains a little bite, but is not chalky in the middle.

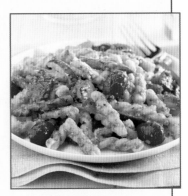

Gemelli and Grilled Summer Vegetables, pg. 239

ANSWERS: Every correct answer is letter "c."

Tofu and Friends

Sometimes tofu, seitan and tempeh are referred to as meat substitutes. It's true that these ingredients can be made into shapes that resemble meat and they have a satisfying chew and somewhat meaty flavor. However, many vegetarians enjoy them because they are delicious and nutritious in and of themselves.

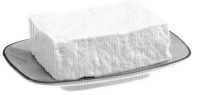

You probably know that tofu is made from soybeans, but you may be unaware that the process that produces it is very similar to making cheese. A salt- or acid-based coagulant is added to soymilk to form curds and whey. (Remember Little Miss Muffet?) Once the curds are drained and pressed you have a block of tofu. While tofu is a relatively recent addition to American kitchens, it has been a huge part of Asian cuisine for centuries.

Buying and Storing Tofu

Tofu comes in many forms as a visit to any Asian market will illustrate, but there are two main types. *Regular or brick tofu* (sometimes called *Chinese tofu*) is sold in the refrigerated section of the supermarket in the produce section or near the dairy case and comes sealed in a plastic tub filled with water. There is usually a choice of soft, medium, firm or extra firm. Once opened, regular tofu will keep in the refrigerator up to 4 days. The water should be drained and replaced daily.

> **Pressing Tofu**
>
> It isn't absolutely necessary, but pressing tofu removes excess moisture, which makes the tofu easier to handle and allows it to absorb flavors better. To press tofu, you need to make a sort of tofu sandwich. Place it on a cutting board or plate lined with a paper towels. Cover with more paper towels and place a flat, heavy object, like a saucepan on top. Press the tofu for 15 minutes or more. Drain excess moisture as needed.

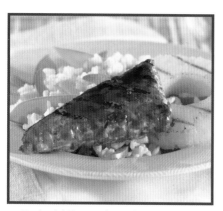

Teriyaki Tempeh with Pineapple, pg. 276

Silken tofu, sometimes called *Japanese tofu*, is the sort that comes in an aseptic box, which does not require refrigeration. While it also comes in soft, medium or firm, the texture of silken tofu is almost custard-like compared to regular. It is an excellent thickener and works well in soups. Silken tofu is too delicate to use in most stir-fries where it will crumble and dissolve.

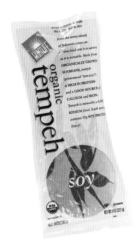

Tempeh

Tempeh (pronounced "tem-pay") is a very nutritious fermented soy food that originated in Indonesia hundreds of years ago. Although it won't win prizes for good looks—it looks like a messy cake of beans and nuts squashed together—tempeh has a nutty, yeasty flavor and chewy texture that is easy to learn to love. You'll find cakes of tempeh, vacuum-packed and refrigerated, in natural food stores and some supermarkets. Soybean tempeh is the classic version, but tempeh can also be made of rice and other grains, or be a mixture of soy and grain.

Using Tempeh

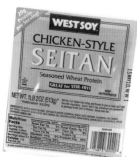

It's best to cook tempeh before eating it, although this is for taste reasons rather than food safety ones. Cooking improves both flavor and texture. Like tofu, tempeh has an ability to readily absorb flavors and cooking enhances this. Its firm texture makes it a great choice to replace ground beef, cook on the grill or use in a sandwich.

Seitan

Seiten (pronounced "say-tan") is sometimes called wheat-meat, gluten-meat or mock duck. It is made from wheat by washing away the starch component until only the wheat protein—gluten— is left. If you've ever eaten mock duck or mock chicken in a Chinese restaurant, you've tried seitan. It is also the base for some commercial vegetarian deli "meats."

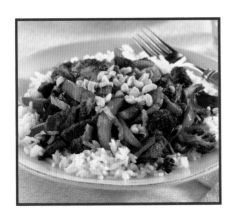

Thai Seitan Stir-Fry, pg. 298

Using Seitan

You'll find seitan in the refrigerated or freezer section of natural food stores packed in a marinade in a tub or a vacuum pack. Varieties are flavored, Asian-style with soy and ginger, or seasoned to taste like chicken or other meat. Seitan is incredibly versatile. It can be stir-fried, baked, broiled or grilled.

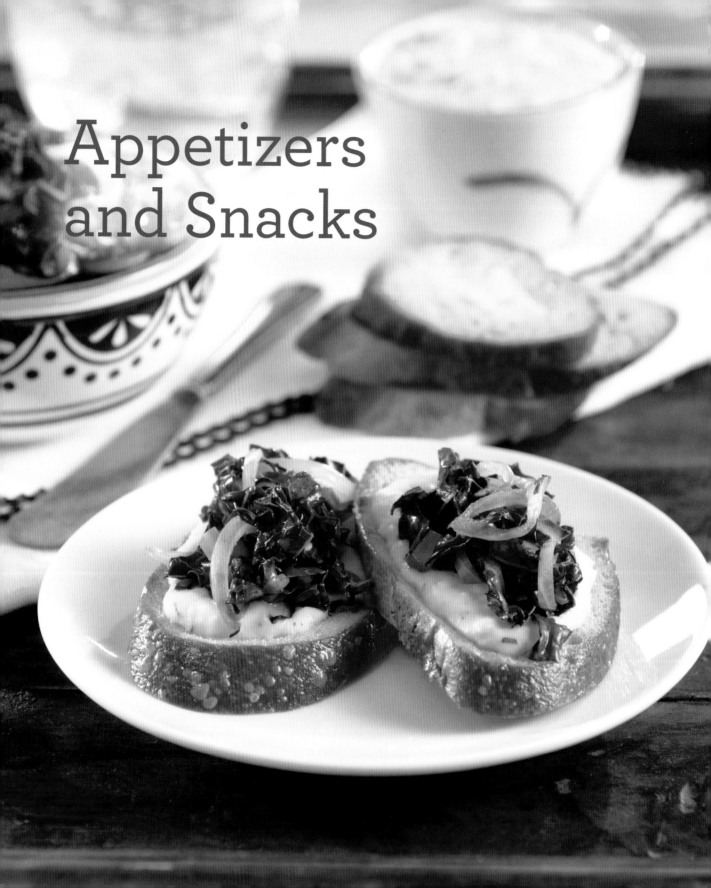

Appetizers and Snacks

Beans and Greens Crostini

4 tablespoons olive oil, divided

1 small onion, thinly sliced

4 cups thinly sliced Italian black kale or other dinosaur kale variety

2 tablespoons minced garlic, divided

1 tablespoon balsamic vinegar

2 teaspoons salt, divided

¼ teaspoon red pepper flakes

1 can (about 15 ounces) cannellini beans, rinsed and drained

1 tablespoon chopped fresh rosemary leaves

Toasted baguette slices

1. Heat 1 tablespoon oil in large skillet over medium heat. Add onion; cook and stir 5 minutes or until softened. Add kale and 1 tablespoon garlic; cook and stir 15 minutes or until kale is softened and most of liquid has evaporated. Stir in vinegar, 1 teaspoon salt and red pepper flakes.

2. Meanwhile, combine beans, remaining 3 tablespoons oil, 1 tablespoon garlic, 1 teaspoon salt and rosemary in food processor; process until smooth.

3. Spread baguette slices with bean mixture; top with kale.

Makes about 24 crostini

Vegetable Empanadas

  2 tablespoons olive oil

  1 cup frozen diced hash brown potatoes

  1 onion, chopped

  1 red bell pepper, chopped

  1 green bell pepper, chopped

  1 package (8 ounces) sliced mushrooms

  2 teaspoons minced garlic

1½ teaspoons ground cumin

½ teaspoon salt

½ teaspoon ground nutmeg

½ teaspoon black pepper

¼ teaspoon ground red pepper

  1 package (17 ounces) frozen puff pastry sheets (2 sheets), thawed

½ cup (2 ounces) shredded Monterey Jack cheese

  3 tablespoons milk

     Salsa

1. Heat oil in large nonstick skillet over medium heat. Add potatoes, onion, bell peppers, mushrooms, garlic, cumin, salt, nutmeg, black pepper and red pepper; cook and stir 5 minutes. Cool to room temperature.

2. Preheat oven to 400°F. Unfold pastry sheets on floured surface. Roll each sheet into 12-inch square with lightly floured rolling pin; cut each square into four squares with sharp knife. Place about ¼ cup filling in corner of each square; sprinkle with 1 tablespoon cheese.

3. Brush small amount of milk on edges of pastry squares. Fold one corner over filling to opposite corner to form triangle; press edges with fork to seal. Cut small slit in top of each triangle with knife. Place triangles on ungreased baking sheets; brush tops with remaining milk.

4. Bake 15 to 20 minutes or until puffed and golden brown. Serve with salsa.

Makes 8 servings

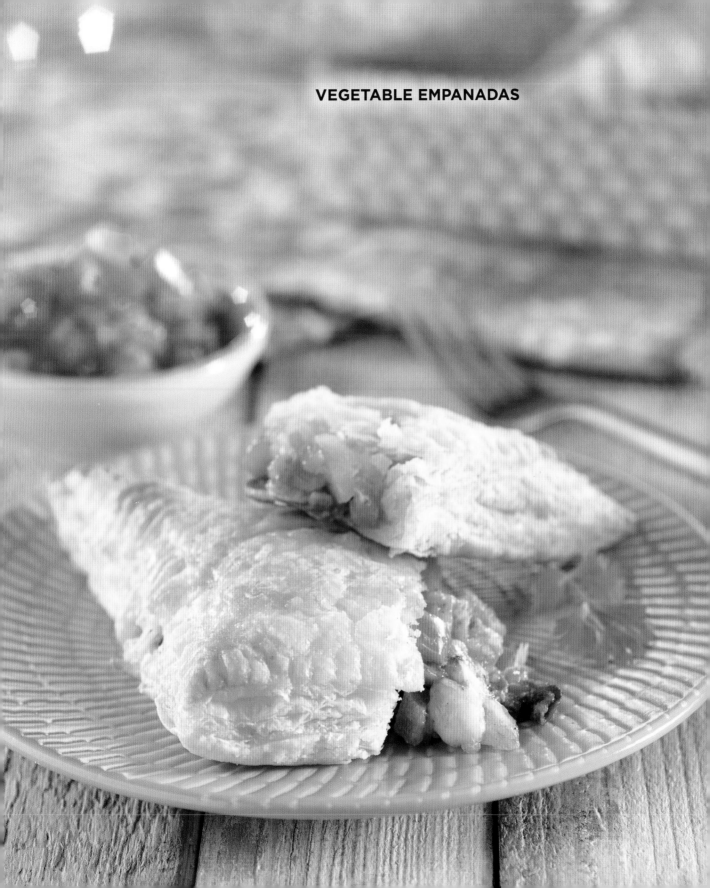

Vegetarian Summer Rolls

1 package (14 ounces) firm tofu, drained

3½ ounces thin rice noodles (rice vermicelli)

½ cup soy sauce, divided

2 tablespoons lime juice

1 tablespoon sugar

2 cloves garlic, minced

1 teaspoon rice vinegar

1 teaspoon dark sesame oil

1 tablespoon vegetable oil

2 medium portobello mushrooms, cut into thin strips

1 tablespoon sesame seeds

12 rice paper wrappers*

1 bunch fresh mint

½ cup shredded carrots

1 yellow bell pepper, cut into thin strips

* Rice paper is a thin, edible wrapper used in Southeast Asian cooking. It is available at specialty stores or Asian markets.

1. Cut tofu crosswise into two pieces, each about 1 inch thick. Arrange between paper towel-lined cutting boards. Place weighted saucepan or baking dish on top; let stand 30 minutes to drain.

2. Place rice noodles in medium bowl; cover with hot water. Soak 20 to 30 minutes or until softened. Drain and cut into 3-inch lengths.

3. Meanwhile, prepare dipping sauce. Combine ¼ cup soy sauce, lime juice, sugar, garlic and vinegar in small bowl; stir until sugar is dissolved. Set aside.

4. Cut tofu into narrow strips about ¼ inch thick. Place in medium bowl with remaining ¼ cup soy sauce and sesame oil; toss gently to coat. Heat vegetable oil in large skillet over medium heat. Add tofu and mushrooms; cook and stir until browned. Sprinkle with sesame seeds.

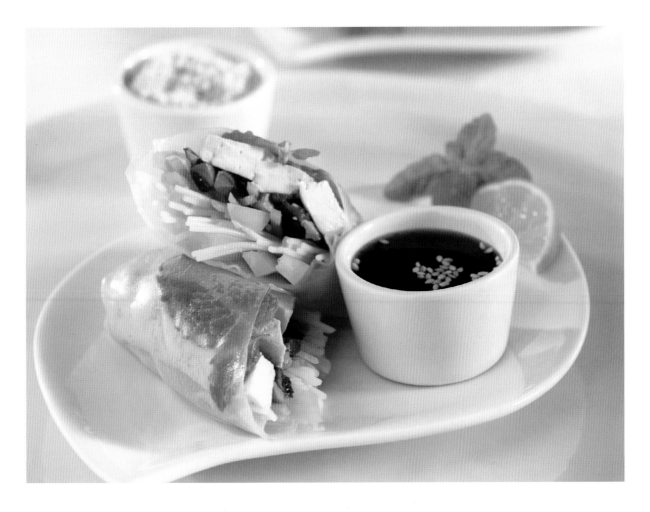

5. Soften rice paper wrappers, one at a time, in bowl of warm water 20 to 30 seconds. Remove from water and place on flat surface lined with clean dish towel. Arrange mint leaves in center of wrapper. Layer with tofu, mushrooms, carrots, noodles and bell pepper.

6. Fold bottom of wrapper up over filling; fold in each side and roll up. Repeat with remaining wrappers. Wrap finished rolls individually in plastic wrap or cover with damp towel until ready to serve to prevent drying out. Serve with dipping sauce.

Makes 12 summer rolls

Fried Tofu with Sesame Dipping Sauce

- 3 tablespoons soy sauce or tamari
- 2 tablespoons unseasoned rice vinegar
- 2 teaspoons sugar
- 1 teaspoon sesame seeds, toasted*
- 1 teaspoon dark sesame oil
- ⅛ teaspoon red pepper flakes
- 1 package (14 ounces) extra firm tofu
- 2 tablespoons all-purpose flour
- 1 egg
- ¾ cup panko bread crumbs
- 4 tablespoons vegetable oil

To toast sesame seeds, spread seeds in small skillet. Shake skillet over medium-low heat about 3 minutes or until seeds begin to pop and turn golden.

1. Whisk soy sauce, vinegar, sugar, sesame seeds, sesame oil and red pepper flakes in small bowl until well blended; set aside.

2. Drain tofu and press between paper towels to remove excess water. Cut crosswise into four slices; cut each slice diagonally into triangles. Place flour in shallow dish. Beat egg in shallow bowl. Place panko in another shallow bowl.

3. Dip each piece of tofu in flour, turning to lightly coat all sides. Dip in egg, letting excess drip back into bowl. Roll in panko to coat.

4. Heat 2 tablespoons vegetable oil in large nonstick skillet over high heat. Reduce heat to medium; add half of tofu in single layer. Cook 1 to 2 minutes per side or until golden brown. Repeat with remaining vegetable oil and tofu. Serve with sauce for dipping.

Makes 4 servings

Variation: To make this recipe vegan, omit the egg. Instead, stir ¼ cup rice milk or plain soymilk into 1 tablespoon cornstarch in small bowl until smooth. Dip floured tofu into the rice milk mixture and proceed with the recipe as directed.

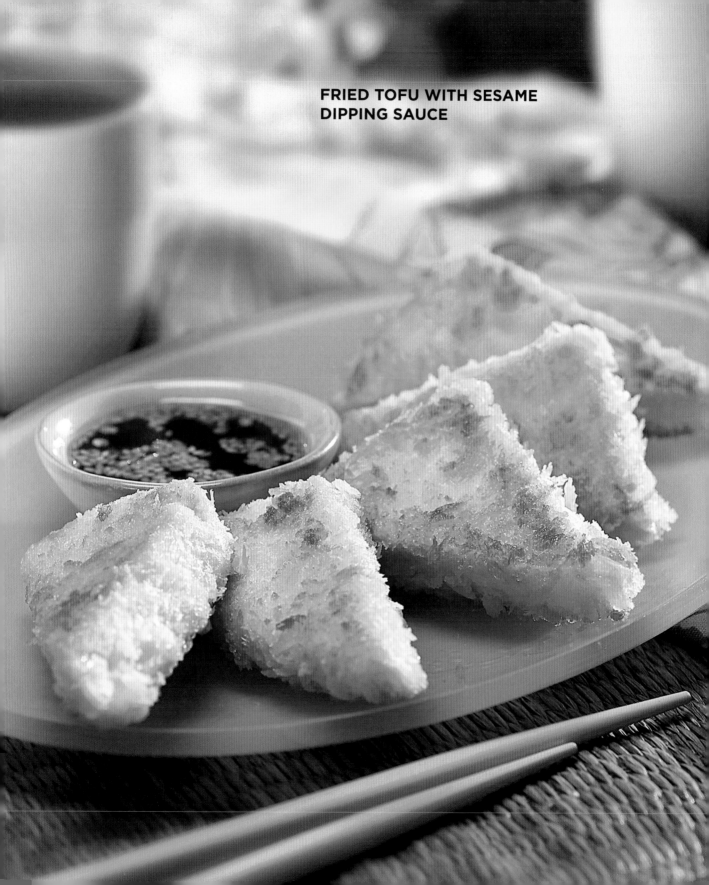

FRIED TOFU WITH SESAME DIPPING SAUCE

Spinach-Cheese Pull-Aparts

 4 tablespoons (½ stick) butter, melted, divided

12 frozen white dinner rolls (⅓ of 3-pound package),* thawed according to package directions

 1 package (10 ounces) frozen chopped spinach, thawed and squeezed dry

 4 green onions, finely chopped (about ¼ cup packed)

 1 clove garlic, minced

 1 teaspoon dried dill weed

 ½ teaspoon salt

 ⅛ teaspoon black pepper

 1 cup (4 ounces) crumbled feta cheese

 ¾ cup (3 ounces) grated Monterey Jack cheese, divided

*If frozen dinner rolls are not available, substitute one 1-pound loaf frozen bread dough or pizza dough. Thaw according to package directions and divide into 12 pieces.

1. Brush large (10-inch) ovenproof skillet with ½ tablespoon butter. Cut each roll in half to make 24 balls of dough.

2. Combine spinach, green onions, garlic, dill, salt and pepper in medium bowl; mix well to break apart spinach. Add feta, ½ cup Monterey Jack and remaining 3½ tablespoons butter; mix well.

3. Coat each ball of dough with spinach mixture; arrange in single layer in prepared skillet. Sprinkle any remaining spinach mixture over and between balls of dough. Cover and let rise in warm place about 40 minutes or until almost doubled in size. Preheat oven to 350°F.

4. Sprinkle remaining ¼ cup Monterey Jack over dough. Bake 35 to 40 minutes or until golden brown. Serve warm.

Makes 24 rolls

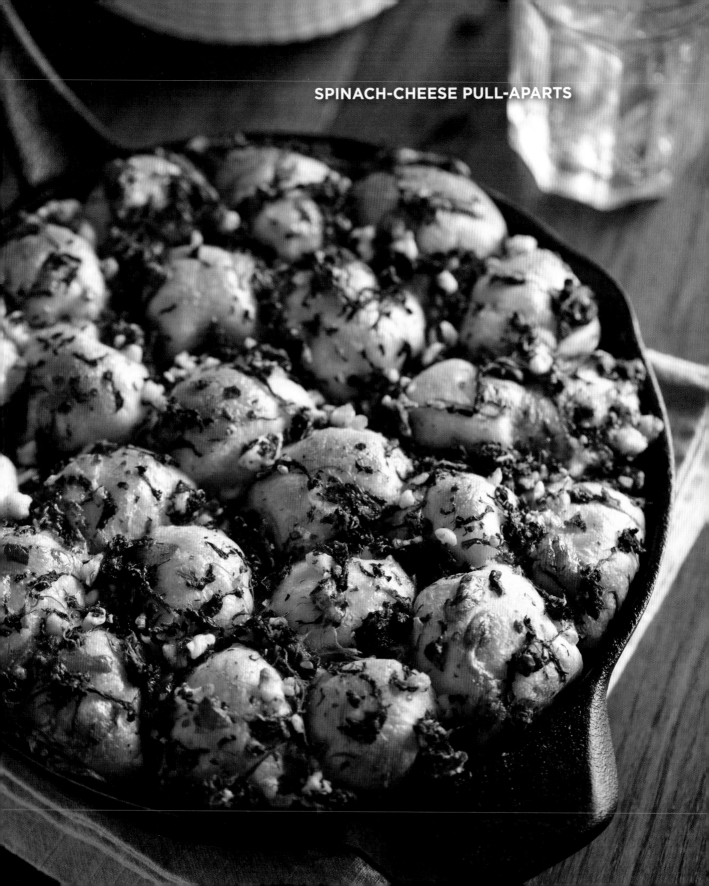

Nicole's Cheddar Crisps

1¾ cups all-purpose flour

½ cup yellow cornmeal

¾ teaspoon sugar

¾ teaspoon salt

½ teaspoon baking soda

½ cup (1 stick) butter, cut into small pieces

1½ cups (6 ounces) shredded sharp Cheddar cheese

½ cup cold water

2 tablespoons white vinegar

Coarsely ground black pepper

1. Combine flour, cornmeal, sugar, salt and baking soda in large bowl. Cut in butter with pastry blender or two knives until mixture resembles coarse crumbs. Stir in cheese, water and vinegar with fork until mixture forms soft dough. Cover and refrigerate 1 hour or freeze 30 minutes or until firm.

2. Preheat oven to 375°F. Line two baking sheets with parchment paper or spray with nonstick cooking spray.

3. Divide dough into four pieces. Roll each piece into paper-thin circle, about 13 inches in diameter, on floured surface. Sprinkle with pepper; press pepper firmly into dough. Cut each circle into eight wedges; place on prepared baking sheets.

4. Bake about 10 minutes or until crisp. Store in airtight container up to 3 days.

Makes 32 crisps

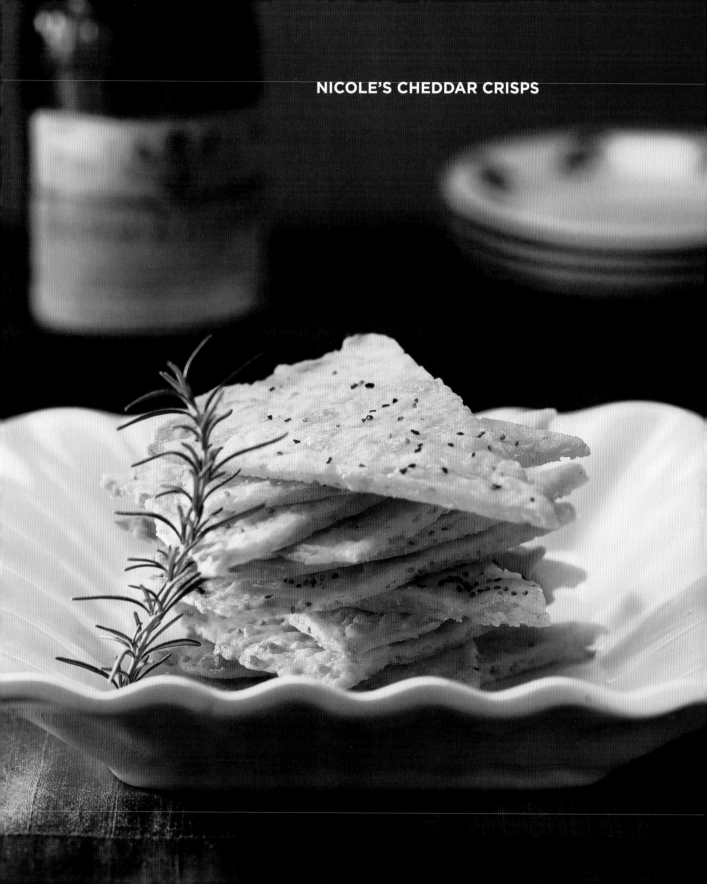

Savory Corn Cakes

    2 cups all-purpose flour
    1 teaspoon baking powder
    ½ teaspoon salt
    2 cups frozen corn, thawed
    1 cup (4 ounces) shredded smoked Cheddar cheese
    1 cup milk
    2 egg whites, beaten
    1 whole egg, beaten
    4 green onions, finely chopped
    2 cloves garlic, minced
    1 tablespoon chili powder
       Salsa (optional)

1. Combine flour, baking powder and salt in large bowl. Add corn, cheese, milk, egg whites, egg, green onions, garlic and chili powder; stir until well blended.

2. Spray large nonstick skillet with nonstick cooking spray; heat over medium-high heat.

3. Drop batter by ¼ cupfuls into skillet. Cook 3 minutes per side or until golden brown. Serve with salsa, if desired.

Makes 12 cakes

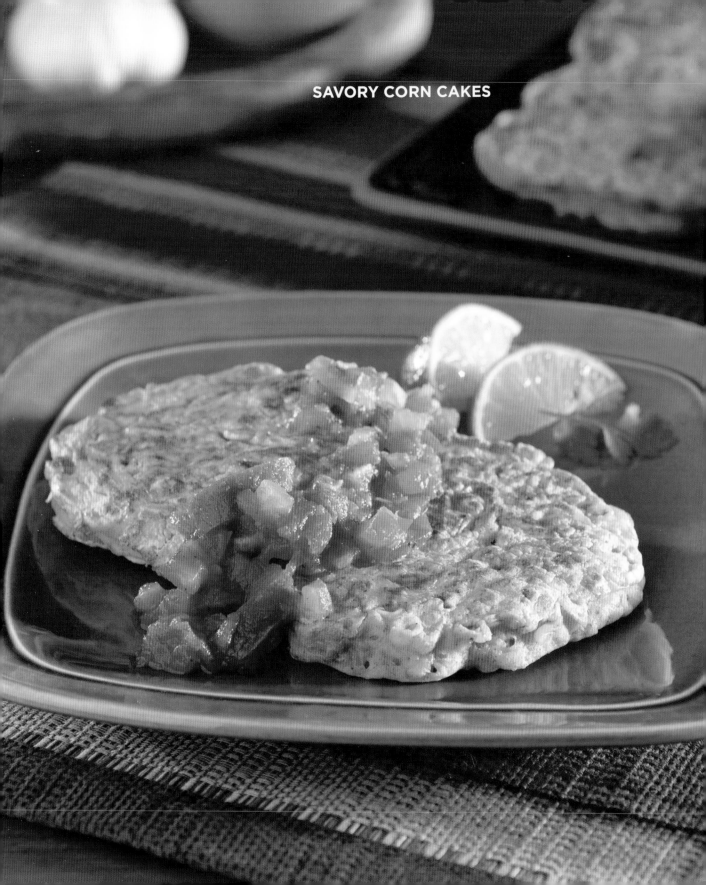

Spicy Polenta Cheese Bites

3 cups water

1 cup corn grits or cornmeal

½ teaspoon salt

¼ teaspoon chili powder

1 tablespoon butter

¼ cup minced onion or shallot

1 tablespoon minced jalapeño pepper*

½ cup (2 ounces) shredded sharp Cheddar or fontina cheese

Jalapeño peppers can sting and irritate the skin, so wear rubber gloves when handling peppers and do not touch your eyes.

1. Spray 8-inch square baking pan with nonstick cooking spray. Bring water to a boil in large nonstick saucepan over high heat. Gradually add grits, stirring constantly. Reduce heat to low; cook and stir until grits are tender and water is absorbed. Stir in salt and chili powder. Remove from heat.

2. Melt butter in small skillet over medium-high heat. Add onion and jalapeño; cook and stir 3 to 5 minutes or until tender. Stir into grits; mix well. Spread in prepared pan. Let stand 1 hour or until cool and firm.

3. Preheat broiler. Cut polenta into 16 squares. Arrange squares on nonstick or foil-lined baking sheet; sprinkle with cheese.

4. Broil 4 inches from heat source 5 minutes or until cheese is melted and slightly browned. Cut squares in half. Serve warm or at room temperature.

Makes 32 appetizers

Tip: For a spicier flavor, add ⅛ teaspoon red pepper flakes to the onion mixture.

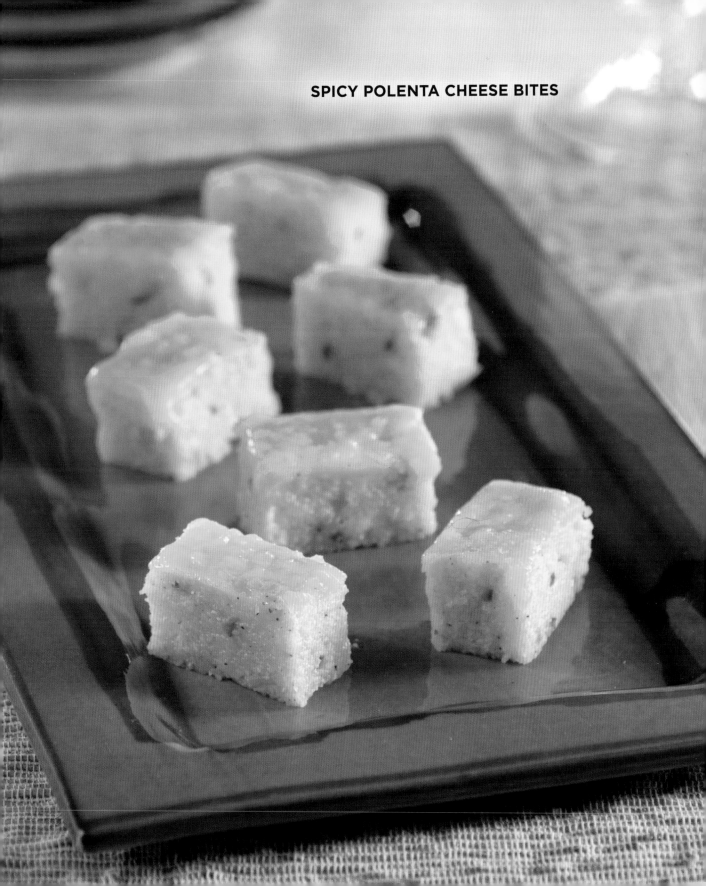

SPICY POLENTA CHEESE BITES

Artichokes with Lemon-Tarragon Butter

     6 cups water
    2¼ teaspoons salt, divided
     2 whole artichokes, stems cut off and leaf tips trimmed
     ¼ cup (½ stick) butter
     ¼ teaspoon grated lemon peel
     2 tablespoons lemon juice
     ¼ teaspoon dried tarragon

1. Bring water and 2 teaspoons salt to a boil in large saucepan over high heat. Add artichokes; return to a boil. Reduce heat to medium-low; cover and simmer 35 to 45 minutes or until leaves detach easily.

2. Turn artichokes upside down to drain well. Cut artichokes in half; use spoon to remove fuzzy choke at base of each artichoke.

3. Combine butter, lemon peel, lemon juice, tarragon and remaining ¼ teaspoon salt in small saucepan; heat over low heat until butter is melted. Serve in small bowls for dipping.

Makes 2 servings

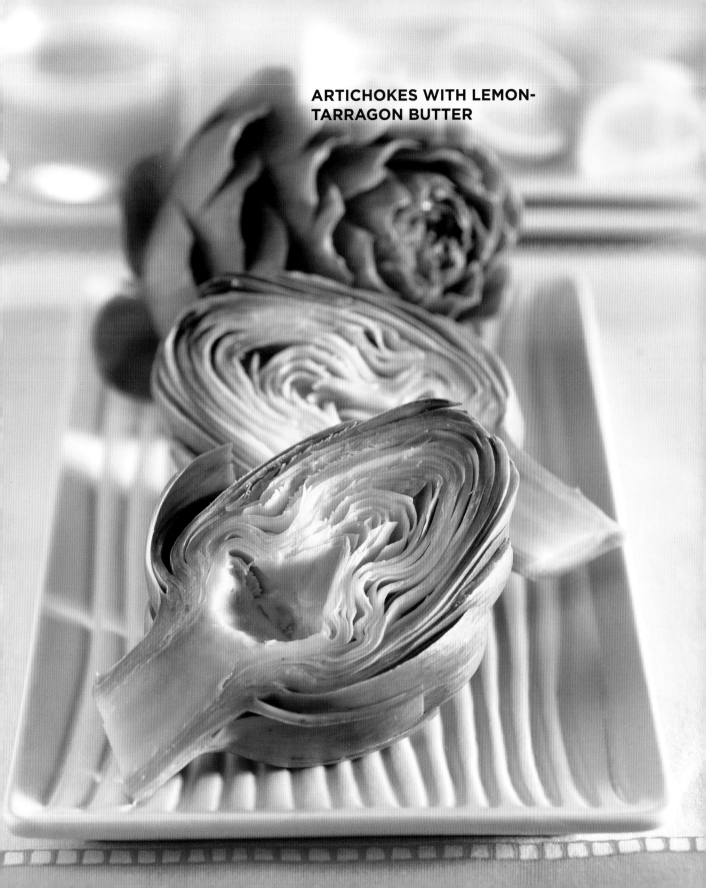

ARTICHOKES WITH LEMON-TARRAGON BUTTER

Socca (Niçoise Chickpea Pancake)

   1 **cup chickpea flour**

   ¾ **teaspoon salt**

   ½ **teaspoon black pepper**

   1 **cup water**

   5 **tablespoons olive oil, divided**

  1½ **teaspoons minced fresh basil** *or* **½ teaspoon dried basil**

   1 **teaspoon minced fresh rosemary leaves** *or* **¼ teaspoon dried rosemary**

   ¼ **teaspoon dried thyme**

1. Sift chickpea flour into medium bowl. Stir in salt and pepper. Gradually whisk in water until smooth. Stir in 2 tablespoons oil. Let stand at least 30 minutes.

2. Preheat oven to 450°F. Place 9- or 10-inch cast iron skillet in oven to heat.

3. Add basil, rosemary and thyme to batter; whisk until smooth. Carefully remove skillet from oven. Add 2 tablespoons oil to skillet, swirling to coat pan evenly. Immediately pour in batter.

4. Bake 12 to 15 minutes or until edge of pancake begins to pull away from side of pan and center is firm. Remove from oven. Preheat broiler.

5. Brush with remaining 1 tablespoon oil. Broil 2 to 4 minutes or until dark brown in spots. Cut into wedges. Serve warm.

Makes 6 servings

Note: To make a thinner, softer crêpe, just increase the amount of water in the recipe by about ¼ cup and cook in batches in a skillet.

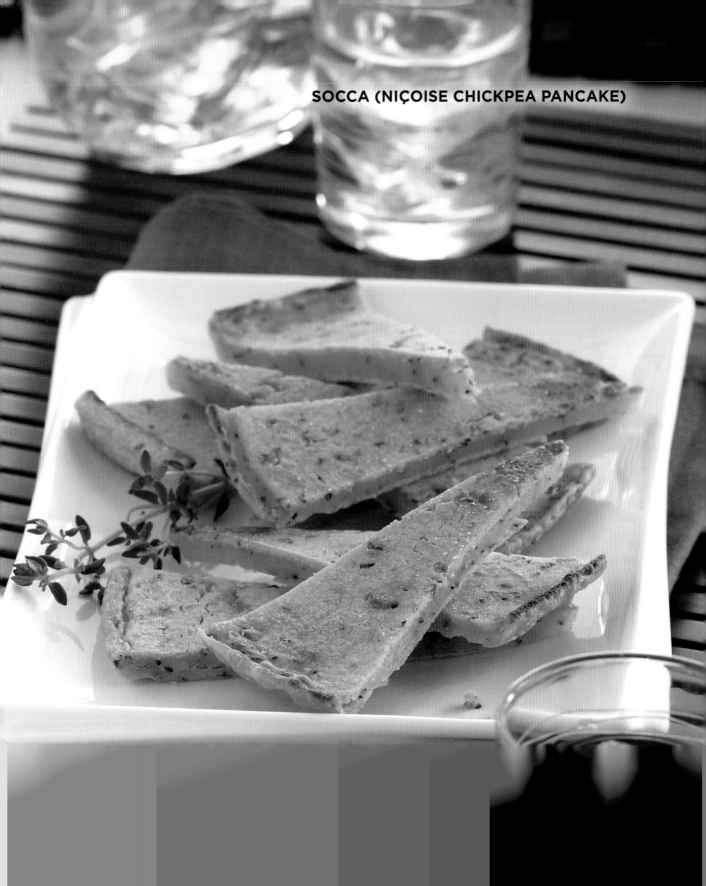
SOCCA (NIÇOISE CHICKPEA PANCAKE)

Edamame Hummus

    1 package (16 ounces) frozen shelled edamame, thawed

    2 green onions, coarsely chopped (about ½ cup)

    ½ cup loosely packed fresh cilantro

    3 to 4 tablespoons water

    2 tablespoons canola oil

    1½ tablespoons lime juice

    1 tablespoon honey

    2 cloves garlic

    1 teaspoon salt

    ¼ teaspoon black pepper

       Rice crackers and/or vegetable sticks

1. Combine edamame, green onions, cilantro, 3 tablespoons water, oil, lime juice, honey, garlic, salt and pepper in food processor; process until smooth. Add additional water to thin dip, if necessary.

2. Serve with rice crackers and/or vegetable sticks for dipping. Store in refrigerator up to 4 days.

Makes 2 cups

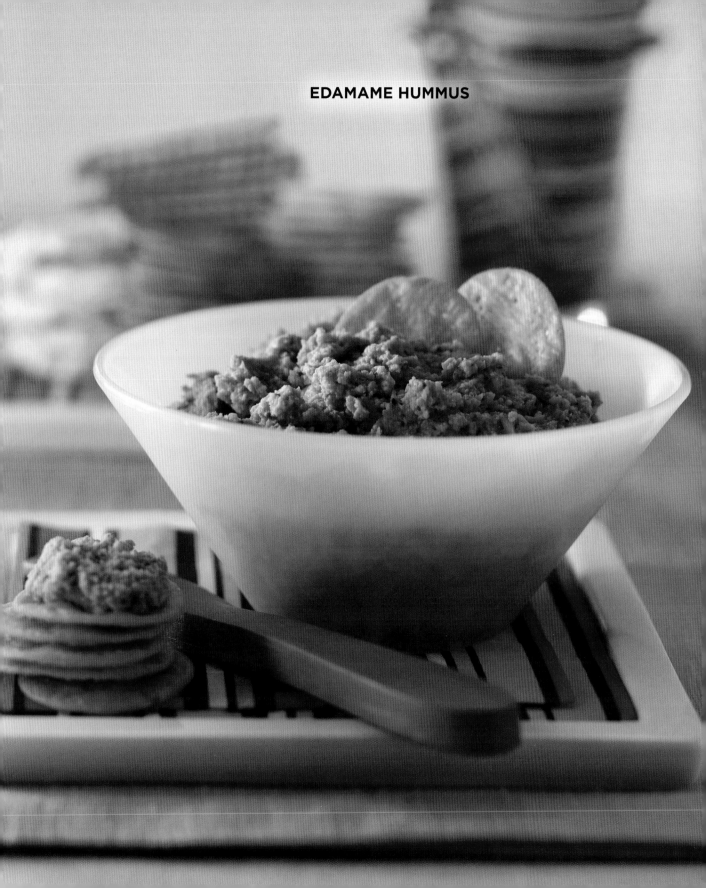

EDAMAME HUMMUS

Light Greek Spanakopita

Olive oil nonstick cooking spray

1 tablespoon olive oil

1 large onion, cut into quarters and sliced

2 cloves garlic, minced

1 package (10 ounces) frozen chopped spinach, thawed and squeezed dry

½ cup (2 ounces) crumbled feta cheese

5 sheets phyllo dough, thawed

2 eggs

¼ teaspoon ground nutmeg

¼ to ½ teaspoon black pepper

⅛ teaspoon salt

1. Preheat oven to 375°F. Spray 8-inch square baking pan with cooking spray.

2. Heat oil in large skillet over medium heat. Add onion; cook and stir 7 to 8 minutes or until soft. Add garlic; cook and stir 30 seconds. Add spinach and cheese; cook and stir until spinach is heated through. Remove from heat.

3. Place one sheet of phyllo dough on counter with long side toward you. (Cover remaining sheets with damp towel until needed.) Spray right half of phyllo with cooking spray; fold left half over sprayed half. Place in prepared pan. (Two edges will hang over sides of pan.) Spray top of phyllo with cooking spray. Spray and fold two more sheets of phyllo the same way. Place sheets in pan at 90 degree angles so edges hang over all four sides of pan. Spray each sheet after placing in pan.

4. Beat eggs, nutmeg, pepper and salt in small bowl. Stir into spinach mixture until well blended. Spread filling over phyllo in pan. Spray and fold one sheet phyllo as above; place over filling, tucking ends under filling. Bring all overhanging edges of phyllo over top sheet; spray lightly wtih cooking spray. Spray and fold last sheet as above; place over top sheet, tucking ends under. Spray lightly.

5. Bake 25 to 27 minutes or until top is lightly browned. Let stand 10 to 15 minutes before serving.

Makes 4 servings

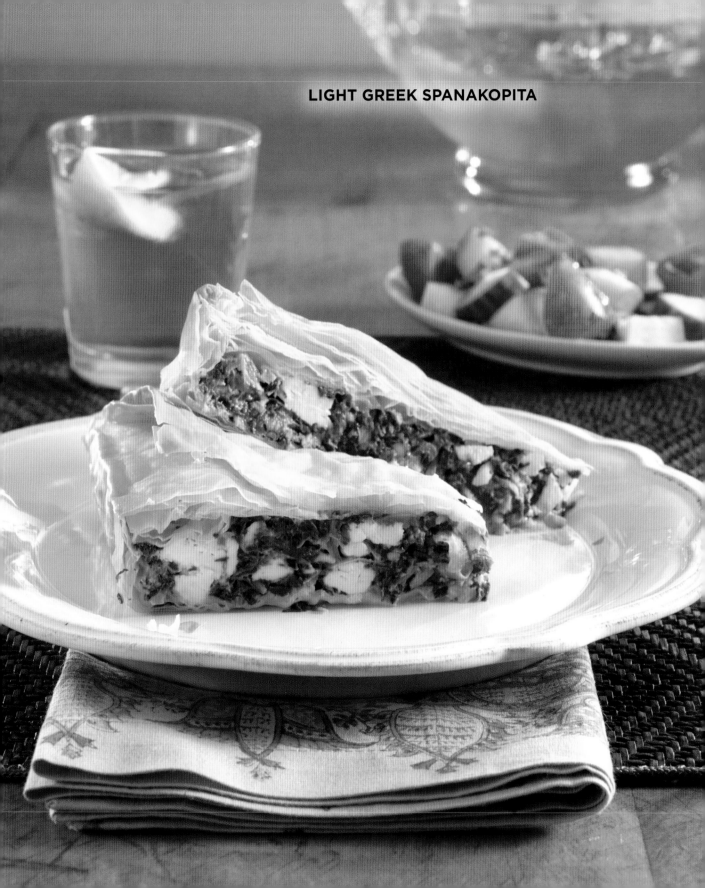

LIGHT GREEK SPANAKOPITA

Tamales

1 package dried corn husks (8 husks)

4 ounces quesadilla cheese or mozzarella cheese

1 can (about 7 ounces) pickled jalapeños

1 can (about 15 ounces) yellow corn, drained, liquid reserved

1 cup plus 3 tablespoons cornmeal

2 tablespoons butter, softened

1 teaspoon salt

Salsa, pico de gallo or guacamole (optional)

1. Soak corn husks in warm water 1 hour or until softened.

2. Cut cheese into 4-inch-long strips. Cut jalapeños into strips. Tear narrow strips of corn husk to use as ties for tamales, if desired.

3. Combine corn and 2 tablespoons reserved corn liquid in food processor; pulse until paste forms. Add 1 cup cornmeal, butter and salt; pulse 1 minute or until dough forms. Add remaining cornmeal gradually until dough is soft and moist but not sticky. Place dough on work surface; keep covered to prevent drying out.

4. Pat corn husk dry. Place 2 tablespoons cornmeal mixture in center of husk. Pat dough into rectangle about 4×2 inches. Arrange one strip of cheese and one strip of jalapeño in center of dough.

5. Lift sides of husk to enclose filling in dough and wrap gently around tamale. Fold bottom of husk over tamale; tie closed with strip of husk or kitchen string. Tie top closed or leave open. Place tamales in steamer basket.

6. Fill large saucepan with water to a depth that will not touch bottom of steamer basket. Bring to a boil. Place steamer basket over water; cover and steam 45 minutes to 1 hour or until tamale no longer sticks to corn husk, adding additional water to saucepan as needed.

7. Serve tamales with salsa, if desired. Tamales may also be refrigerated or frozen and reheated in steamer or microwave.

Makes 8 tamales

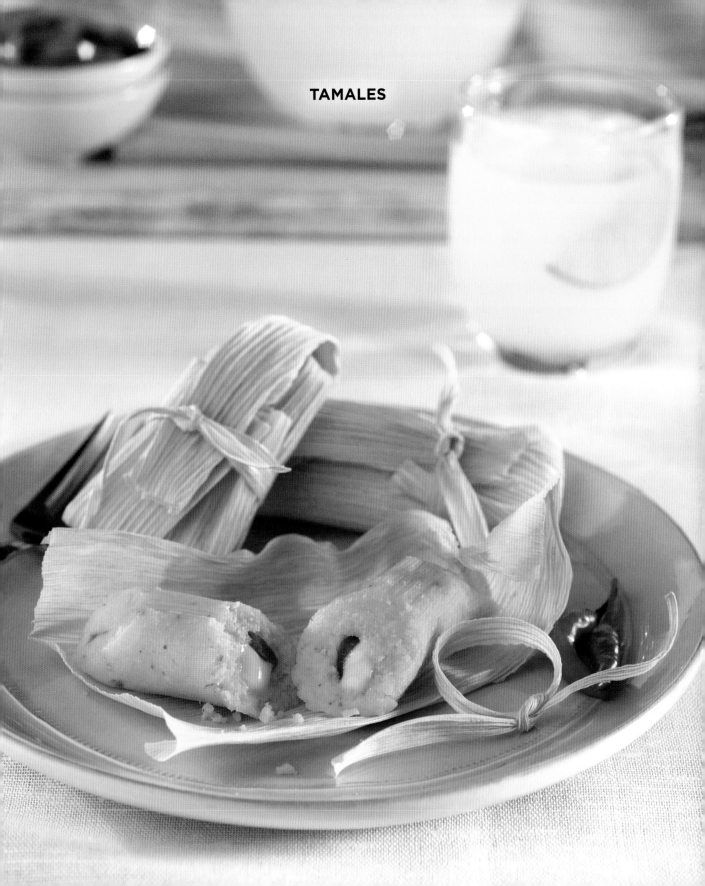

TAMALES

Beer Batter Tempura

1½ cups all-purpose flour

1½ cups Japanese beer, chilled

1 teaspoon salt

Dipping Sauce (recipe follows)

Vegetable oil for frying

½ pound green beans or asparagus tips

1 large sweet potato, cut into ¼-inch slices

1 medium eggplant, cut into ¼-inch slices

1. Combine flour, beer and salt in medium bowl just until mixed. Batter should be thin and lumpy. *Do not overmix.* Let stand 15 minutes.

2. Meanwhile, prepare Dipping Sauce; set aside.

3. Heat 1 inch of oil in large saucepan to 375°F; adjust heat to maintain temperature.

4. Dip 10 to 12 green beans in batter; add to hot oil. Fry until light golden brown. Remove to wire racks or paper towels to drain; keep warm. Repeat with remaining vegetables, working with only one vegetable at a time and being careful not to crowd vegetables. Serve with Dipping Sauce.

Makes 4 servings

Dipping Sauce: Combine ½ cup soy sauce, 2 tablespoons rice wine, 1 tablespoon sugar and ½ teaspoon white vinegar in small saucepan; cook and stir over medium heat 3 minutes or until sugar dissolves. Add 2 teaspoons minced fresh ginger and 1 clove minced garlic; cook and stir 2 minutes. Stir in 2 thinly sliced green onions; remove from heat.

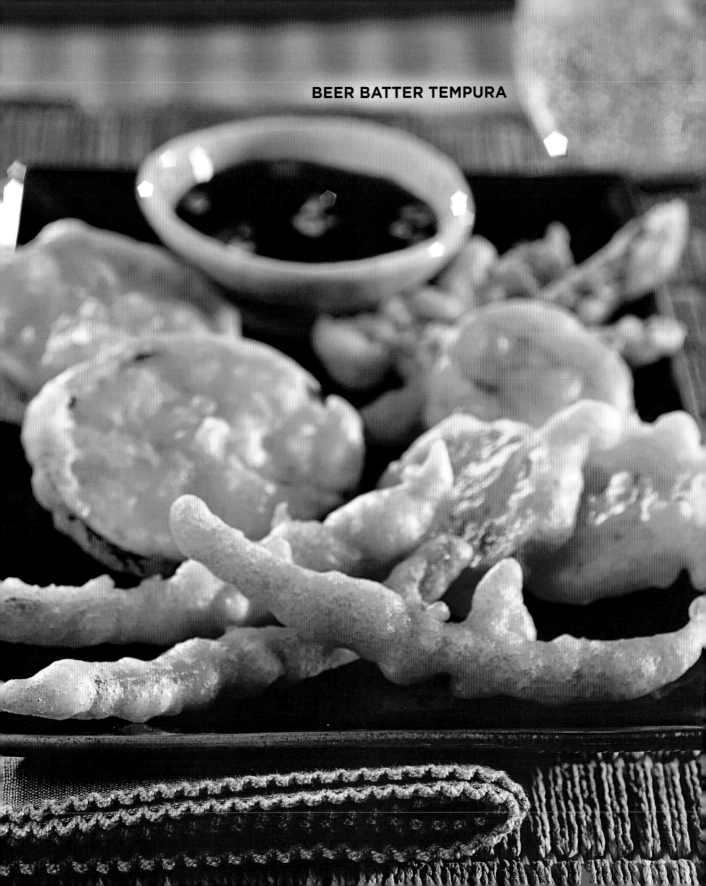

BEER BATTER TEMPURA

Fabulous Feta Frittata

  8 eggs

 ¼ cup plain Greek yogurt

 ¼ cup chopped fresh basil

 ¼ teaspoon salt

 ¼ teaspoon black pepper

  1 tablespoon olive oil or butter

  1 package (4 ounces) crumbled feta cheese with basil, olives
     and sun-dried tomatoes *or* 1 cup crumbled plain feta cheese

 ¼ cup pine nuts (optional)

1. Preheat broiler. Beat eggs, yogurt, basil, salt and pepper in medium bowl until well blended.

2. Heat oil in large ovenproof skillet over medium heat, tilting skillet to coat bottom and side. Pour egg mixture into skillet; cover and cook 8 to 10 minutes or until eggs are set around edge (center will be wet).

3. Sprinkle with cheese and pine nuts, if desired. Transfer to broiler; broil 4 to 5 inches from heat source 2 minutes or until center is set and pine nuts are golden brown.

Makes 4 servings

Tip: This frittata also makes a great meal. Cut it into quarters and serve it hot with fruit for breakfast, tuck a wedge into half a pita for lunch, or serve it alongside roasted red potatoes for dinner.

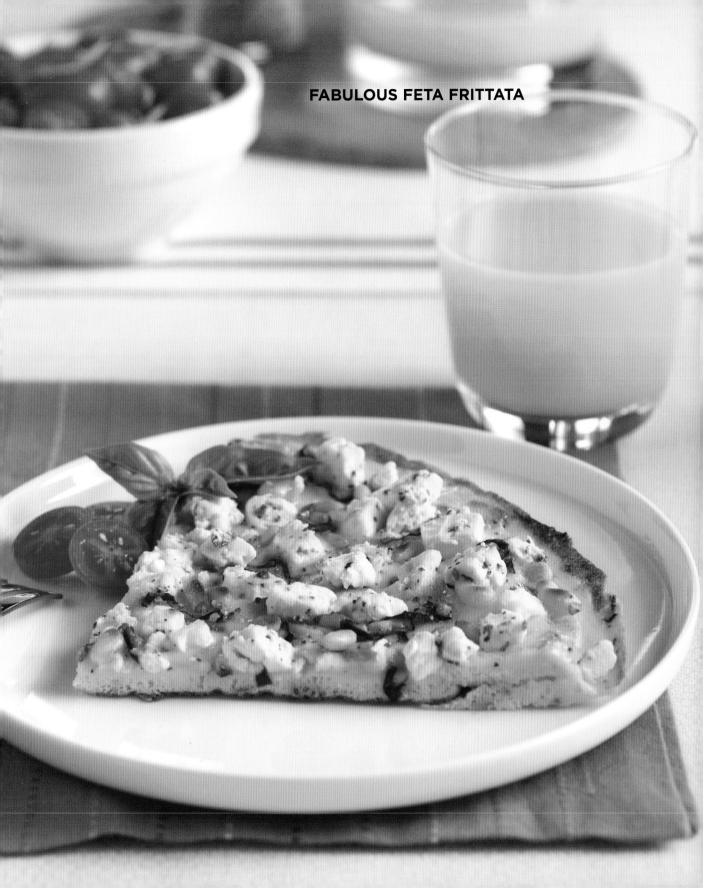

Avocado Lime Ice Cream

    4 cups milk
    1 cup sugar
    3 egg yolks
    4 ripe avocados
       Juice and peel of 2 limes

1. Combine milk and sugar in medium saucepan; cook and stir over medium-high heat just until milk begins to boil. Remove from heat.

2. Whisk egg yolks in medium bowl. Continue whisking while gradually adding ¼ cup hot milk mixture to egg yolks. Slowly pour egg mixture back into saucepan with remaining milk mixture. Cook over medium heat, whisking slowly until first bubble forms. *Do not boil.*

3. Pour custard mixture into medium bowl; cover and refrigerate 2 hours or until cold.

4. Cut avocados in half; remove pits. Scoop avocado into medium mixer bowl. Add lime peel and juice; beat with electric mixer at medium until smooth. Scrape bowl. Add chilled milk mixture; beat at low speed until blended.*

5. Freeze mixture in ice cream maker according to manufacturer's directions until soft.

6. Transfer ice cream to airtight containers; freeze several hours or until firm. Use within 1 week.

*For smoother ice cream, strain mixture through fine-mesh sieve before freezing.

Makes about 1¹/₂ quarts ice cream

Tip: This creamy, slightly sweet ice cream makes a great accompaniment to your favorite Mexican dishes as a first course or a dessert. It's also a refreshing snack on a summer day.

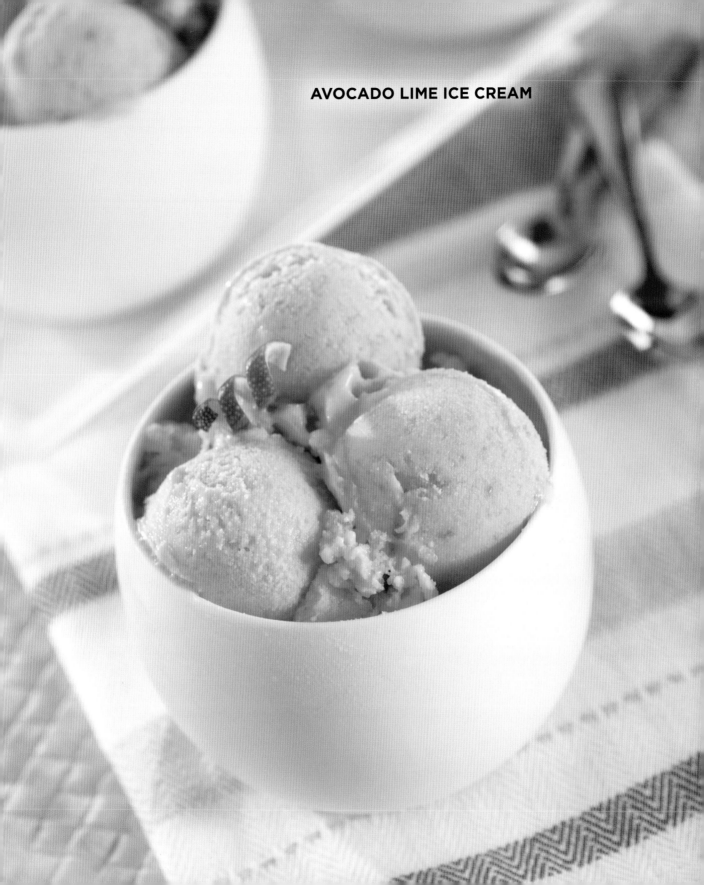
AVOCADO LIME ICE CREAM

Samosas

2¼ cups plus 3 tablespoons all-purpose flour

½ teaspoon salt

3 to 4 cups plus 4 tablespoons vegetable oil, divided

¾ cup warm water

2 large potatoes, peeled

1 bunch green onions, trimmed and chopped

2 fresh green chiles, seeded and minced (optional)

½ cup fresh cilantro, chopped

1 teaspoon whole cumin seeds

2 teaspoons curry powder

½ teaspoon salt

Tamarind Sauce (recipe follows)

1. Combine 2¼ cups flour and salt in bowl of stand mixer; beat at low speed 5 seconds to combine. Add 2 tablespoons oil; beat at low speed until mixture resembles fine bread crumbs. Add ¾ cup warm water; beat 45 seconds or just until dough comes together. Add remaining 3 tablespoons flour; beat 4 minutes or until dough is smooth and elastic. Shape dough into a ball. Place in greased bowl; turn to grease top. Cover and let stand 30 to 40 minutes.

2. Meanwhile, place potatoes in large saucepan; cover with cold water. Bring to a boil over high heat. Reduce heat to low; cover and simmer 20 minutes or until tender. Drain potatoes; let stand until cool enough to handle. Peel and cut into ½-inch pieces.

3. Heat 2 tablespoons oil in large skillet over medium-high heat. Add green onions; cook and stir 45 seconds. Add potatoes, chiles, if desired, cilantro, cumin seeds, curry and salt; cook and stir 1 minute or until fragrant. Set aside to cool.

4. Divide dough into 16 equal pieces; roll into balls. Roll balls into 4-inch circles on floured surface with floured rolling pin. Place 2 heaping teaspoons potato mixture in center of each circle. Lift one side of dough circle; crease in the middle. Lift opposite side of dough; pinch edges together. Fold up bottom end and pinch closed to form triangle. Place samosas on baking sheet; refrigerate 1 hour. Prepare Tamarind Sauce.

5. Heat 2 inches oil in large deep skillet to 360°F over medium heat. Working in batches, fry samosas 1 to 2 minutes per side until golden brown (return oil to 360°F between batches). Drain on paper towel-lined plate. Serve warm with Tamarind Sauce.

Makes 16 samosas

Tamarind Sauce: Combine 2 cups water, ⅓ cup sugar and 2 tablespoons tamarind paste in small saucepan; bring to a boil over medium heat. Reduce heat to low; simmer until reduced by two thirds.

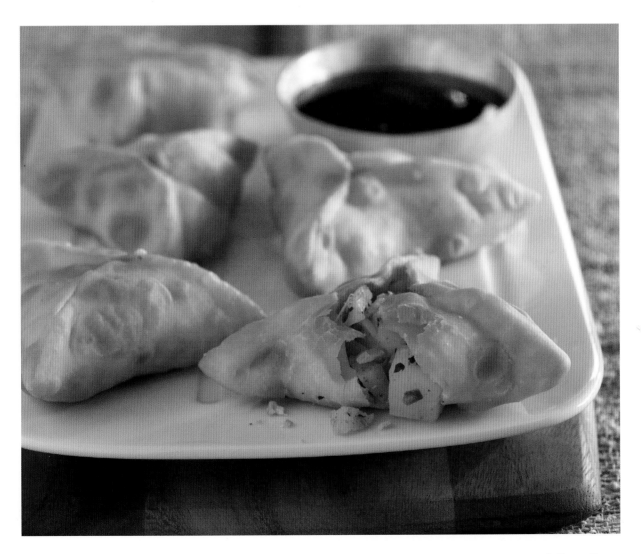

Veggie Sushi Rolls

2 tablespoons unseasoned rice vinegar

1 teaspoon sugar

½ teaspoon salt

2 cups cooked short grain brown rice

4 sheets sushi nori

1 teaspoon toasted sesame seeds

½ English cucumber, cut into ¼-inch thin pieces

½ red bell pepper, cut into ¼-inch thin pieces

½ ripe avocado, cut into ½-inch thin pieces

Pickled ginger and/or wasabi paste (optional)

1. Combine vinegar, sugar and salt in large bowl. Stir in rice until coated. Cover with damp towel until ready to use.

2. Prepare small bowl with water and splash of vinegar to rinse fingers and prevent rice from sticking while working. Place one sheet of nori horizontally on bamboo sushi mat or waxed or parchment paper, rough side up. Using wet fingers, spread about ½ cup rice evenly over nori, leaving 1-inch border along bottom edge. Sprinkle rice with ¼ teaspoon sesame seeds. Place one fourth each of cucumber, bell pepper and avocado on top of rice.

3. Pick up edge of mat nearest you. Roll mat forward, wrapping rice around fillings and pressing gently to form log; press gently to seal. Place roll on cutting board, seam side down. Repeat with remaining nori and fillings.

4. Slice each roll into 6 pieces using sharp knife.* Cut off ends, if desired. Serve with pickled ginger and/or wasabi, if desired.

*Wipe knife with damp cloth between cuts, if necessary.

Makes 24 pieces (about 4 servings)

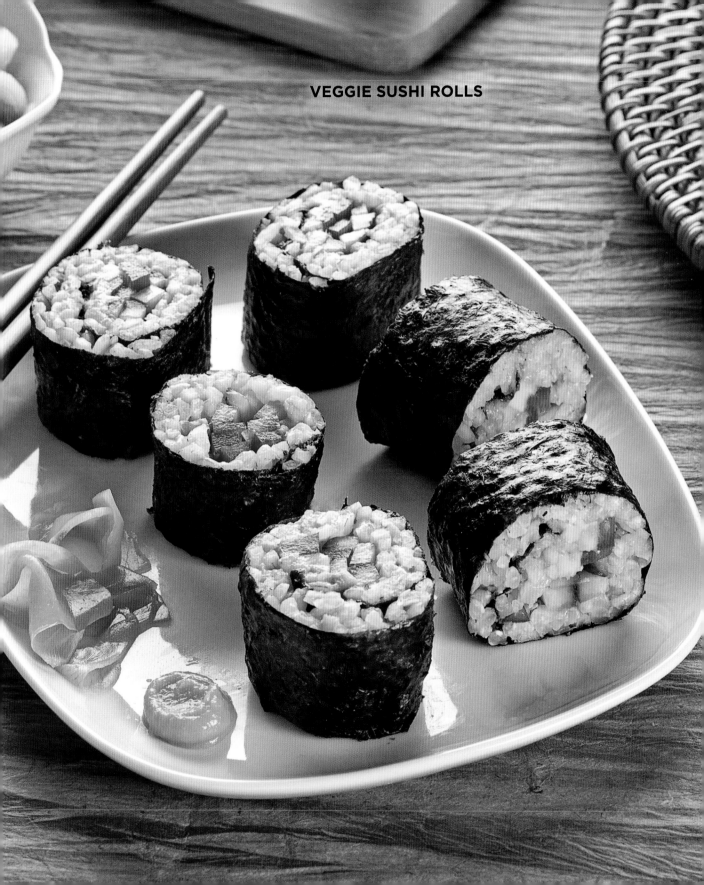

VEGGIE SUSHI ROLLS

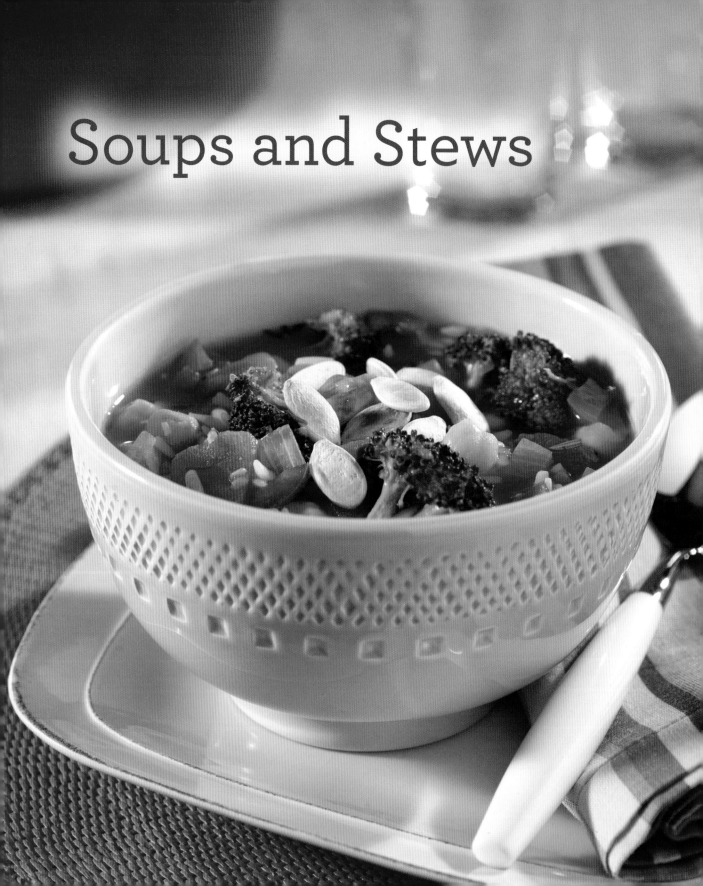

Soups and Stews

Chickpea-Vegetable Soup

    1 tablespoon olive oil
    1 cup chopped onion
    ½ cup chopped green bell pepper
    2 cloves garlic, minced
    2 cans (about 14 ounces each) chopped tomatoes
    3 cups water
    2 cups broccoli florets
    1 can (about 15 ounces) chickpeas, rinsed, drained and slightly mashed
    ½ cup (3 ounces) uncooked orzo or rosamarina pasta
    1 whole bay leaf
    1 tablespoon chopped fresh thyme *or* 1 teaspoon dried thyme
    1 tablespoon chopped fresh rosemary leaves *or* 1 teaspoon dried rosemary
    1 tablespoon lime or lemon juice
    ½ teaspoon salt
    ½ teaspoon ground turmeric
    ¼ teaspoon ground red pepper
    ¼ cup pumpkin seeds or sunflower kernels

1. Heat oil in large saucepan over medium heat. Add onion, bell pepper and garlic; cook and stir 5 minutes or until vegetables are tender.

2. Add tomatoes, water, broccoli, chickpeas, orzo, bay leaf, thyme, rosemary, lime juice, salt, turmeric and red pepper; bring to a boil over high heat. Reduce heat to medium-low; cover and simmer 10 to 12 minutes or until orzo is tender.

3. Remove and discard bay leaf. Sprinkle with pumpkin seeds just before serving.

Makes 4 servings

Lentil Vegetable Stew

    3 tablespoons olive or vegetable oil
    1 large onion, coarsely chopped
    1 can (28 ounces) crushed tomatoes
    2 cups water
    1 tablespoon cider vinegar
    1 tablespoon curry powder
 1½ teaspoons salt
 1½ teaspoons ground cumin
 1½ teaspoons ground coriander
    1 teaspoon ground ginger
 1¼ cups dried lentils, rinsed and sorted*
    2 cups cauliflower florets
    1 cup chopped red bell pepper
    1 cup chopped yellow squash

Packages of dried lentils may contain dirt and tiny stones. Thoroughly rinse lentils, then sort through them and discard any unusual-looking pieces.

1. Heat oil in large saucepan over medium heat. Add onion; cook and stir 5 minutes or until softened.

2. Stir in tomatoes, water, vinegar, curry powder, salt, cumin, coriander and ginger until blended. Stir in lentils; bring to a boil. Reduce heat to medium-low; simmer 35 to 40 minutes or until lentils begin to soften.

3. Add cauliflower, bell pepper and squash; simmer 30 minutes or until vegetables and lentils are tender.

Makes 8 servings

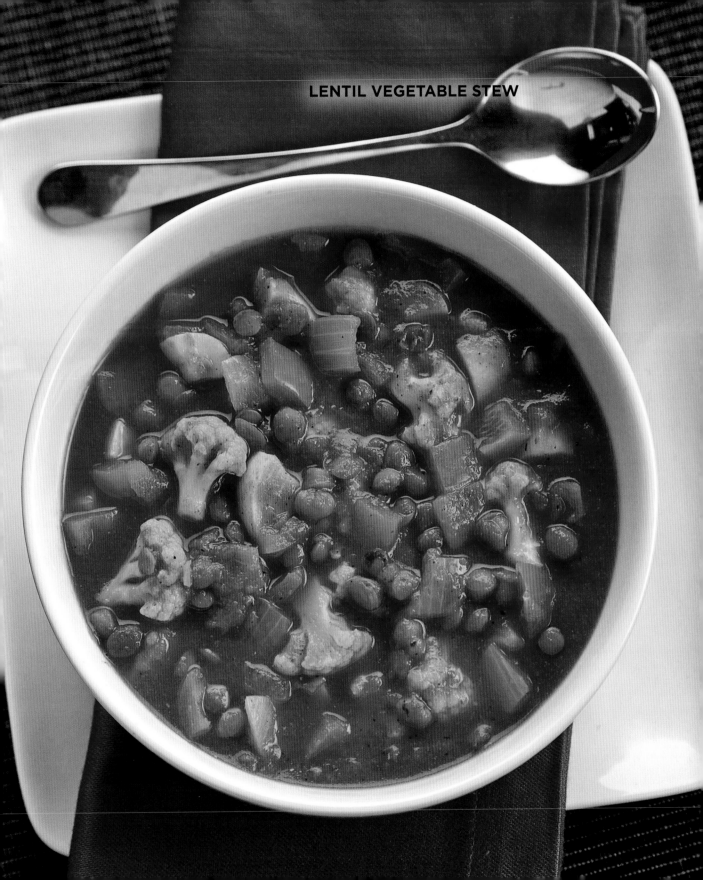

Curried Sweet Potato and Carrot Soup

2 sweet potatoes, peeled and cut into ¾-inch pieces (about 5 cups)

2 cups baby carrots

1 onion, chopped

¾ teaspoon curry powder

½ teaspoon salt

½ teaspoon black pepper

½ teaspoon ground cinnamon

¼ teaspoon ground ginger

4 cups vegetable broth

¾ cup half-and-half

1 tablespoon maple syrup

Candied ginger (optional)

Slow Cooker Directions

1. Combine sweet potatoes, carrots, onion, curry powder, salt, pepper, cinnamon and ground ginger in slow cooker. Stir in broth.

2. Cover; cook on LOW 7 to 8 hours.

3. Working in batches, blend soup in blender or food processor until smooth. Return soup to slow cooker. (Or use hand-held immersion blender.) Stir in half-and-half and maple syrup. Cover; cook on HIGH 15 minutes or until heated through. Garnish with candied ginger.

Makes 8 servings

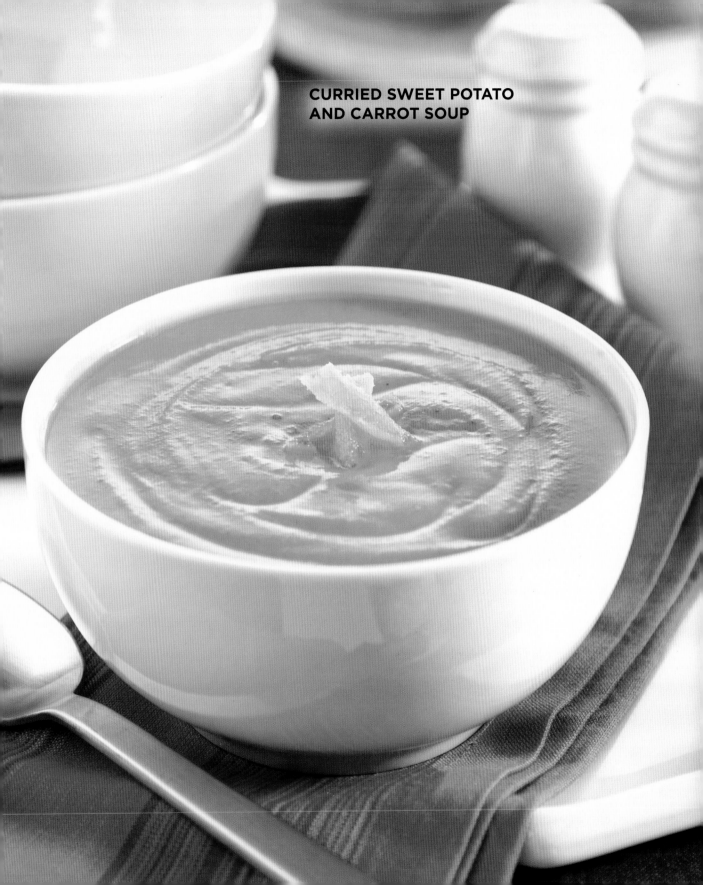

CURRIED SWEET POTATO AND CARROT SOUP

Mediterranean Eggplant and White Bean Stew

  1 tablespoon olive oil

  1 medium onion, chopped

  1 medium eggplant (1 pound), peeled and cut into ¾-inch pieces

  4 cloves garlic, minced

  1 can (28 ounces) stewed tomatoes, undrained

  2 bell peppers (1 red and 1 yellow), cut into ¾-inch pieces

  1 teaspoon dried oregano

  ¼ teaspoon red pepper flakes (optional)

  1 can (about 15 ounces) Great Northern or cannellini beans, rinsed and drained

  6 tablespoons grated Parmesan cheese

  ¼ cup chopped fresh basil

1. Heat oil in large saucepan over medium heat. Add onion; cook and stir 5 minutes. Add eggplant and garlic; cook and stir 5 minutes. Stir in tomatoes, bell peppers, oregano and red pepper flakes, if desired. Reduce heat to medium-low; cover and simmer 20 minutes or until vegetables are tender.

2. Stir in beans; simmer, uncovered, 5 minutes. Sprinkle with cheese and basil.

Makes 6 servings

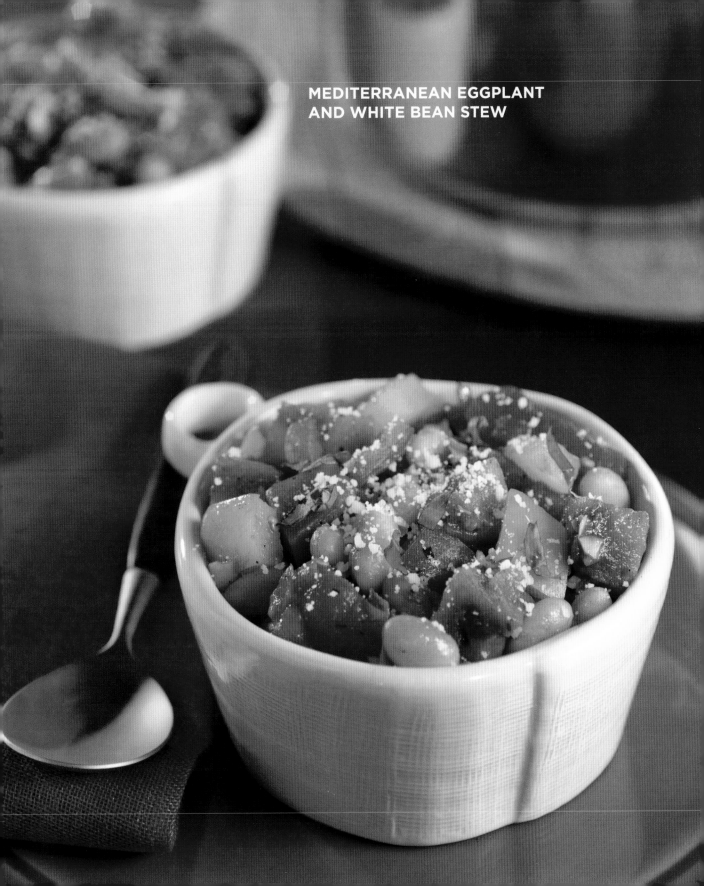

MEDITERRANEAN EGGPLANT
AND WHITE BEAN STEW

Sweet Red Bell Pepper Soup

8 red bell peppers

1 onion, thinly sliced

3 cloves garlic, minced

2 tablespoons olive oil

1 teaspoon black pepper

1 teaspoon dried oregano

2 tablespoons balsamic vinegar

2 teaspoons sugar

Fresh thyme sprigs (optional)

Slow Cooker Directions

1. Cut bell peppers in half; remove stems and seeds. Cut into quarters.

2. Combine bell peppers, onion, garlic, oil, black pepper and oregano in slow cooker; stir to combine.

3. Cover; cook on HIGH 4 hours or until bell peppers are very tender; stirring halfway through cooking time.

4. Purée soup in slow cooker using hand-held immersion blender. Or, transfer mixture in batches to blender or food processor and blend until smooth. Stir in vinegar and sugar. Garnish with thyme.

Makes 8 servings

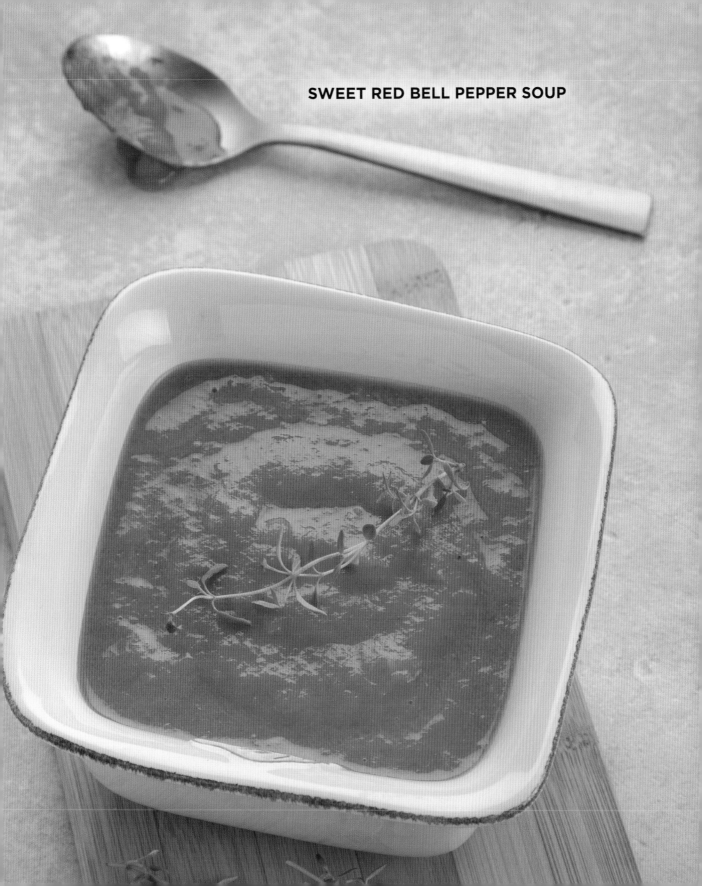

SWEET RED BELL PEPPER SOUP

Barley Stew with Cornmeal-Cheese Dumplings

2 cans (11½ ounces each) spicy vegetable juice cocktail

1 can (about 15 ounces) butter beans or lima beans, rinsed and drained

1 can (about 14 ounces) stewed tomatoes, undrained

1 cup sliced zucchini

1 cup sliced carrots

1 cup water

½ cup chopped peeled parsnip

⅓ cup quick-cooking barley

1 bay leaf

2 tablespoons chopped fresh thyme

1½ tablespoons chopped fresh rosemary leaves

⅓ cup all-purpose flour

⅓ cup cornmeal

1 teaspoon baking powder

¼ cup milk

1 tablespoon canola oil

⅓ cup shredded Cheddar cheese

1. Combine vegetable juice, beans, tomatoes with juice, zucchini, carrots, water, parsnip, barley, bay leaf, thyme and rosemary in large saucepan; bring to a boil over high heat. Reduce heat to medium-low; cover and simmer 20 to 25 minutes or until tender, stirring occasionally. Remove and discard bay leaf.

2. Combine flour, cornmeal and baking powder in medium bowl. Combine milk and oil in small bowl; stir into flour mixture. Stir in cheese until blended.

3. Drop dough by spoonfuls in four mounds onto boiling stew. Cover and simmer 10 to 12 minutes or until toothpick inserted near center of dumplings comes out clean.

Makes 4 servings

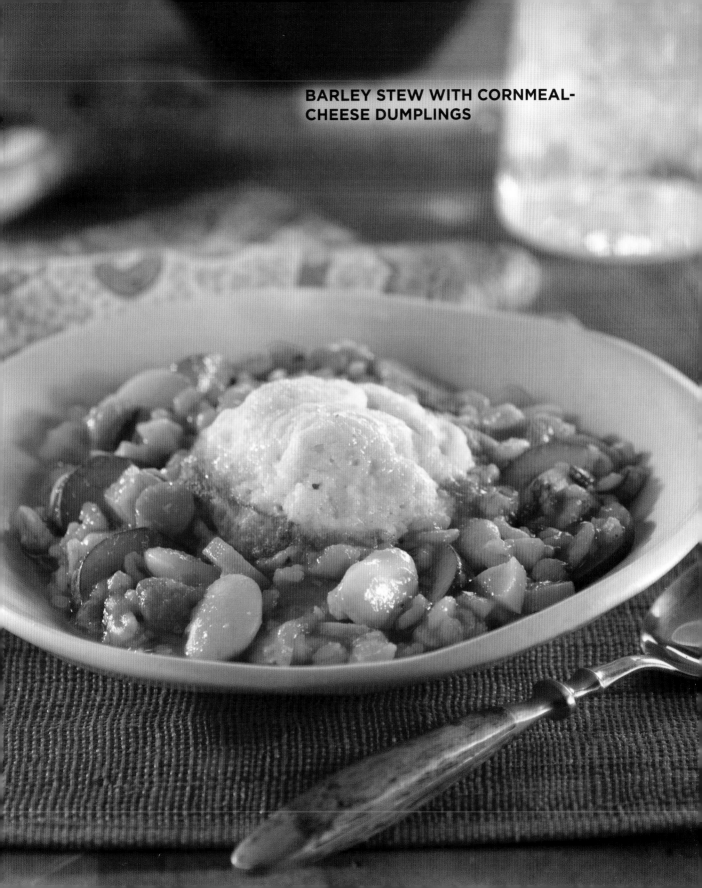

BARLEY STEW WITH CORNMEAL-CHEESE DUMPLINGS

White Bean and Escarole Soup

1½ cups dried baby lima beans, rinsed and sorted

  1 tablespoon olive oil

 ½ cup chopped celery

 ⅓ cup coarsely chopped onion

  2 cloves garlic, minced

  2 cans (about 14 ounces each) whole tomatoes, undrained, chopped

 ½ cup chopped fresh parsley

  2 tablespoons chopped fresh rosemary leaves

 ¼ teaspoon black pepper

  3 cups shredded fresh escarole

1. Place dried beans in large bowl; cover completely with water. Soak 6 to 8 hours or overnight. Drain beans; place in large saucepan or Dutch oven. Cover beans with about 3 cups water; bring to a boil over high heat. Reduce heat to low; cover and simmer about 1 hour or until soft. Drain beans; return to saucepan.

2. Heat oil in medium skillet over medium heat. Add celery, onion and garlic; cook and stir 5 minutes or until onion is tender.

3. Add celery mixture and tomatoes with liquid to beans; bring to a boil over high heat. Stir in parsley, rosemary and pepper. Reduce heat to low; cover and simmer 15 minutes. Add escarole; simmer, uncovered, 5 minutes.

Makes 6 servings

Tip: Store dried lima beans (also known as butter beans) in an airtight container in a cool, dry place for up to 1 year. When soaking, do not allow beans to soak for longer than 12 hours or they may begin to ferment.

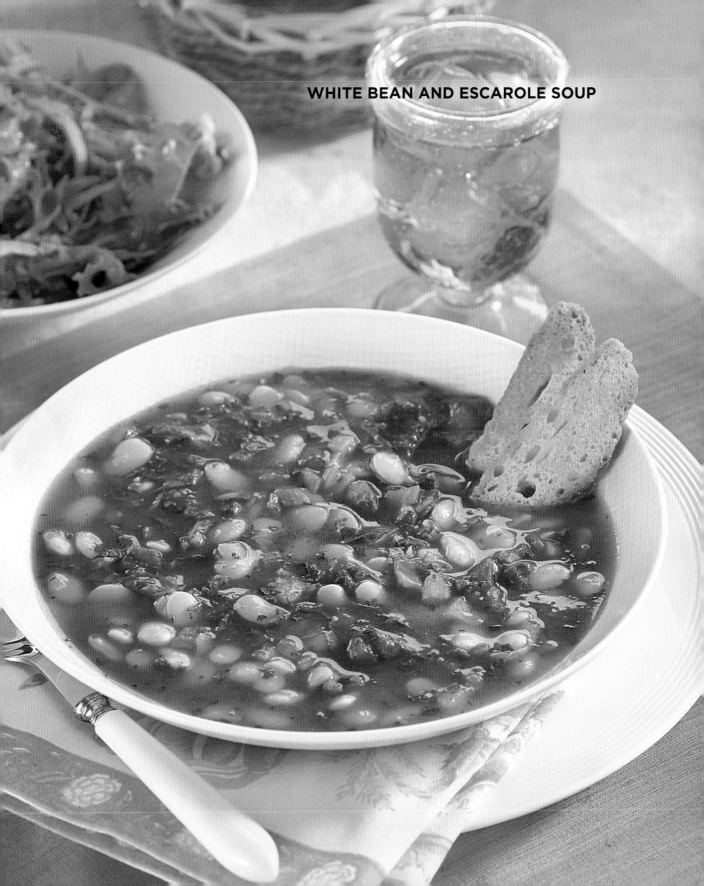

WHITE BEAN AND ESCAROLE SOUP

Chile Pepper and Corn Cream Chowder

 2 tablespoons butter

 1 cup chopped onion

 2 Anaheim or poblano chile peppers,* seeded and diced

 ½ cup thinly sliced celery

 1 package (16 ounces) frozen corn

12 ounces unpeeled new red potatoes, diced

 4 cups whole milk

 6 ounces cream cheese, cubed

 2 teaspoons salt

 ¾ teaspoon black pepper

Anaheim chiles are medium-size green peppers with a long, narrow shape. They are generally mild in flavor, with just a hint of heat and spice.

1. Melt butter in large saucepan over medium-high heat. Add onion, Anaheim peppers and celery; cook and stir 5 minutes or until onion is translucent.

2. Add corn, potatoes and milk; bring to a boil. Reduce heat to medium-low; cover and simmer 10 minutes or until potatoes are tender.

3. Remove from heat; add cream cheese, salt and black pepper. Stir until cream cheese is melted.

Makes 4 to 6 servings

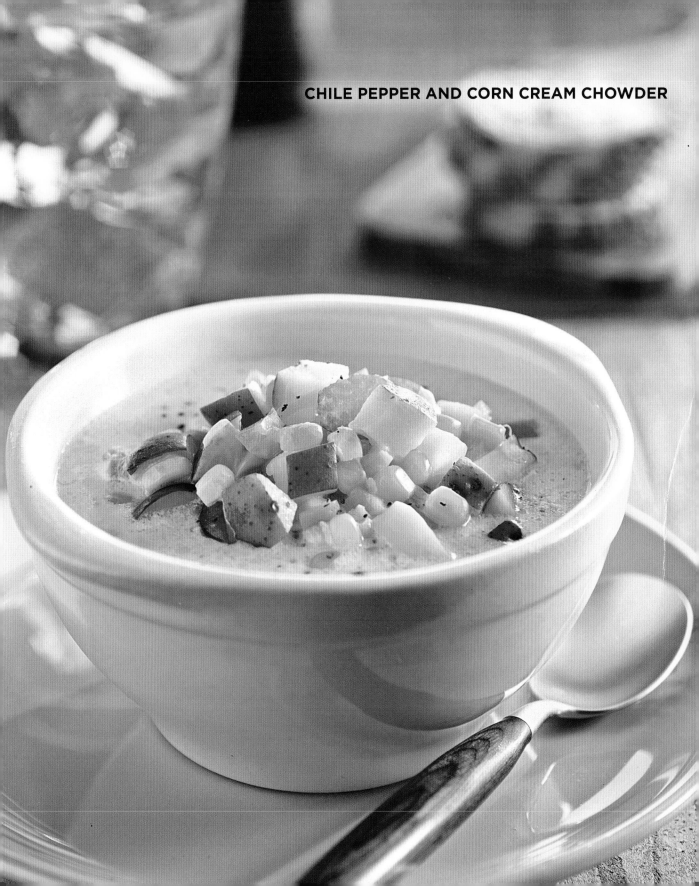

Gazpacho

6 large very ripe tomatoes (about 3 pounds), divided

1½ cups tomato juice

1 clove garlic

2 tablespoons lime juice

2 tablespoons olive oil

1 tablespoon white wine vinegar

1 teaspoon sugar

½ to 1 teaspoon salt

½ teaspoon dried oregano

6 green onions, sliced

¼ cup finely chopped celery

¼ cup finely chopped seeded cucumber

1 to 2 jalapeño peppers, seeded and minced

1 cup diced avocado

1 red or green bell pepper, chopped

Croutons

2 tablespoons chopped fresh cilantro

Lime wedges (optional)

1. Seed and finely chop one tomato; set aside. Coarsely chop remaining five tomatoes; blend half of tomatoes, ¾ cup tomato juice and garlic in blender until smooth. Press through sieve into large bowl; discard seeds. Repeat with remaining coarsely chopped tomatoes and ¾ cup tomato juice.

2. Whisk lime juice, oil, vinegar, sugar, salt and oregano into tomato mixture. Stir in finely chopped tomato, green onions, celery, cucumber and jalapeños. Cover and refrigerate at least 4 hours or up to 24 hours.

3. Stir soup; ladle into chilled bowls. Top with avocado, bell pepper, croutons and cilantro. Serve with lime wedges, if desired.

Makes 4 servings

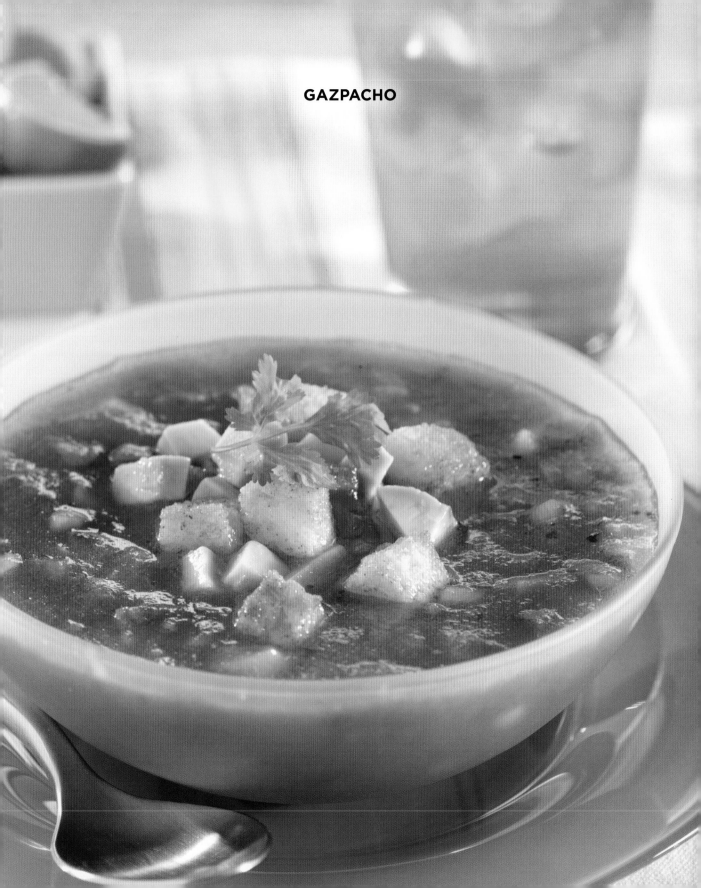
GAZPACHO

Chunky Vegetable Chili

    2 cans (about 15 ounces each) Great Northern beans, rinsed and drained
    1 onion, chopped
    2 stalks celery, diced
    1 carrot, diced
    1 cup frozen corn
    1 cup water
    1 can (6 ounces) tomato paste
    1 can (4 ounces) diced green chiles, undrained
    3 cloves garlic, minced
    1 tablespoon chili powder
    2 teaspoons dried oregano
    ½ teaspoon salt

Slow Cooker Directions

Combine all ingredients in slow cooker. Cover; cook on LOW 5½ to 6 hours or until vegetables are tender.

Makes 6 servings

Serving Suggestion: Serve chili with a sliced toasted baguette, cornbread or warm torillas.

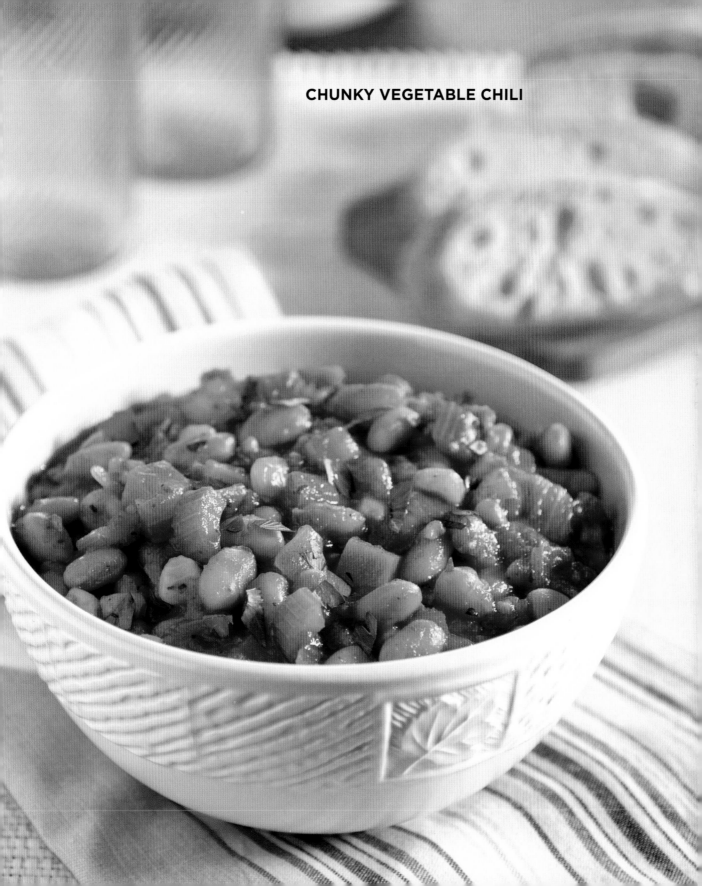

CHUNKY VEGETABLE CHILI

Italian Mushroom Soup

½ cup dried porcini mushrooms (about ½ ounce)

1 tablespoon olive oil

2 cups chopped onions

8 ounces sliced cremini or white mushrooms, plus additional for garnish

2 cloves garlic, minced

¼ teaspoon dried thyme

¼ cup all-purpose flour

4 cups vegetable broth

½ cup whipping cream

⅓ cup Marsala wine (optional)

Salt and black pepper

1. Place dried mushrooms in small bowl; cover with boiling water. Let stand 15 minutes or until tender.

2. Meanwhile, heat oil in large saucepan over medium heat. Add onions; cook 6 minutes or until translucent, stirring occasionally. Add cremini mushrooms, garlic and thyme; cook 8 minutes, stirring occasionally. Reserve several mushrooms for garnish, if desired. Add flour; cook and stir 1 minute. Stir in broth.

3. Drain porcini mushrooms, reserving liquid. Strain soaking liquid. Chop porcini mushrooms; add to saucepan with strained liquid. Bring to a boil. Reduce heat to medium-low; simmer 10 minutes.

4. Working in batches, blend soup in blender or food processor until smooth. Return soup to saucepan. (Or use hand-held immersion blender.) Stir in cream and Marsala, if desired; season with salt and pepper. Simmer over medium-low heat 5 minutes or until heated through. Garnish with reserved mushrooms.

Makes 6 to 8 servings

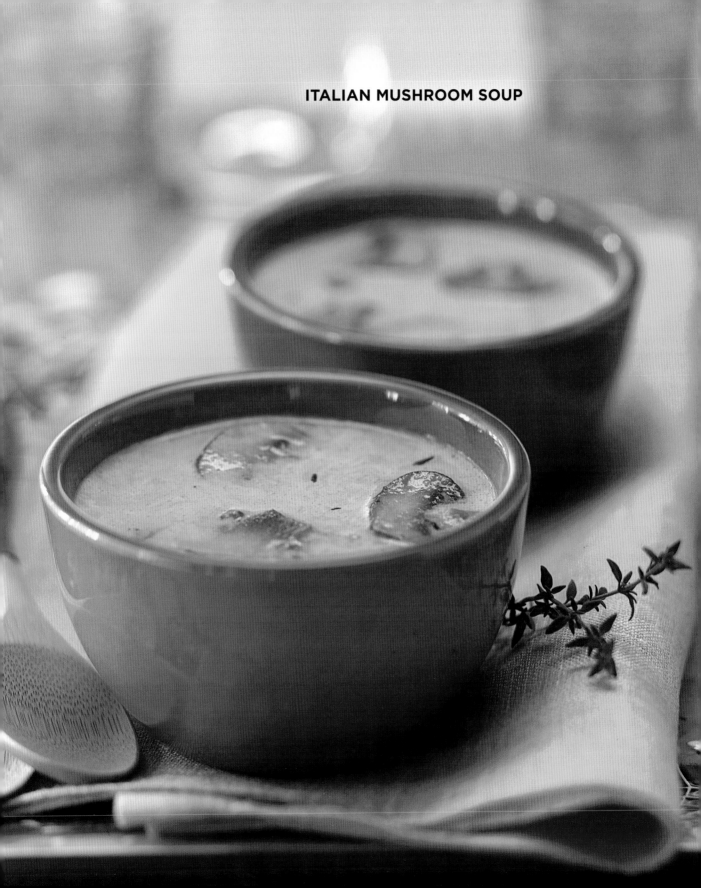

ITALIAN MUSHROOM SOUP

Lentil and Spinach Stew

1 tablespoon olive oil

3 medium stalks celery, cut into ½-inch pieces

3 medium carrots, cut into ½-inch pieces

1 medium onion, chopped

3 cloves garlic, minced

4 cups vegetable broth

1 can (about 14 ounces) diced tomatoes

1 cup dried brown lentils, rinsed and sorted*

2 teaspoons ground cumin

½ teaspoon dried basil

½ teaspoon salt

¼ teaspoon black pepper

5 cups baby spinach

3 cups hot cooked ditalini pasta

*Packages of dried lentils may contain dirt and tiny stones. Thoroughly rinse lentils, then sort through them and discard any unusual-looking pieces.

Slow Cooker Directions

1. Heat oil in large skillet over medium-high heat. Add celery, carrots, onion and garlic; cook and stir 3 to 4 minutes or until vegetables begin to soften.

2. Spray inside of slow cooker with nonstick cooking spray. Transfer vegetable mixture to slow cooker. Stir in broth, tomatoes, lentils, cumin, basil, salt and pepper.

3. Cover; cook on LOW 8 to 9 hours or until lentils are tender but still hold their shape.

4. Stir in spinach just before serving. Serve over pasta.

Makes 4 servings

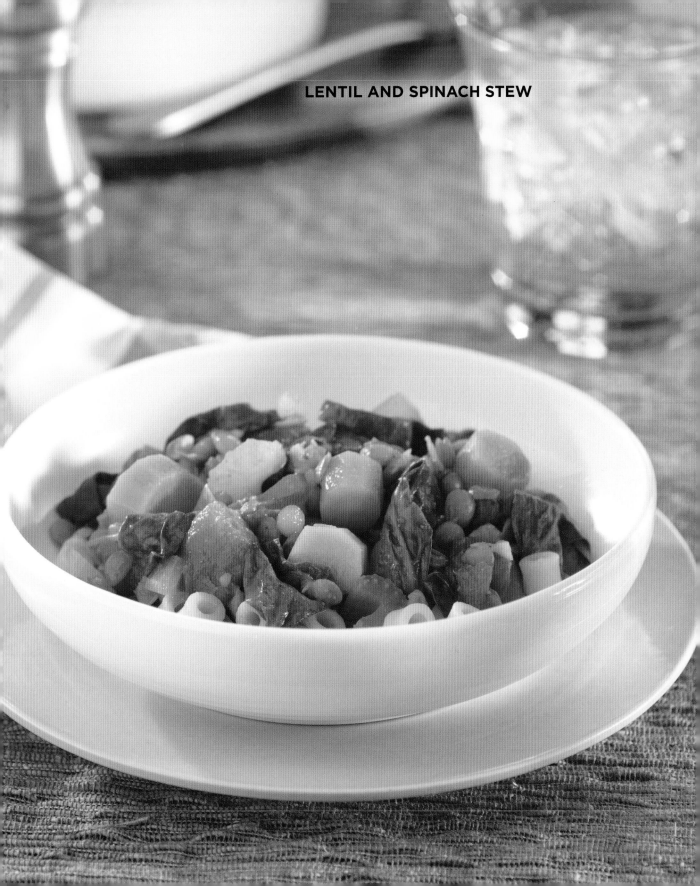

Hot and Sour Soup with Bok Choy and Tofu

  1 tablespoon dark sesame oil

  4 ounces shiitake mushrooms, stems finely chopped, caps thinly sliced

  2 cloves garlic, minced

  2 cups mushroom or vegetable broth

  1 cup plus 2 tablespoons cold water, divided

  2 tablespoons reduced-sodium soy sauce

1½ tablespoons rice vinegar or white wine vinegar

  ¼ teaspoon red pepper flakes

1½ tablespoons cornstarch

  2 cups coarsely chopped bok choy leaves or napa cabbage

10 ounces silken extra firm tofu, well drained, cut into ½-inch cubes

  1 green onion, thinly sliced

1. Heat oil in large saucepan over medium heat. Add mushrooms and garlic; cook and stir 3 minutes. Add broth, 1 cup water, soy sauce, vinegar and red pepper flakes; bring to a boil. Reduce heat to medium-low; simmer, uncovered, 5 minutes.

2. Whisk remaining 2 tablespoons water into cornstarch in small bowl until smooth. Stir into soup; simmer 2 minutes or until thickened.

3. Stir in bok choy; simmer 2 to 3 minutes or until wilted. Stir in tofu; heat through. Sprinkle with green onion.

Makes 4 servings

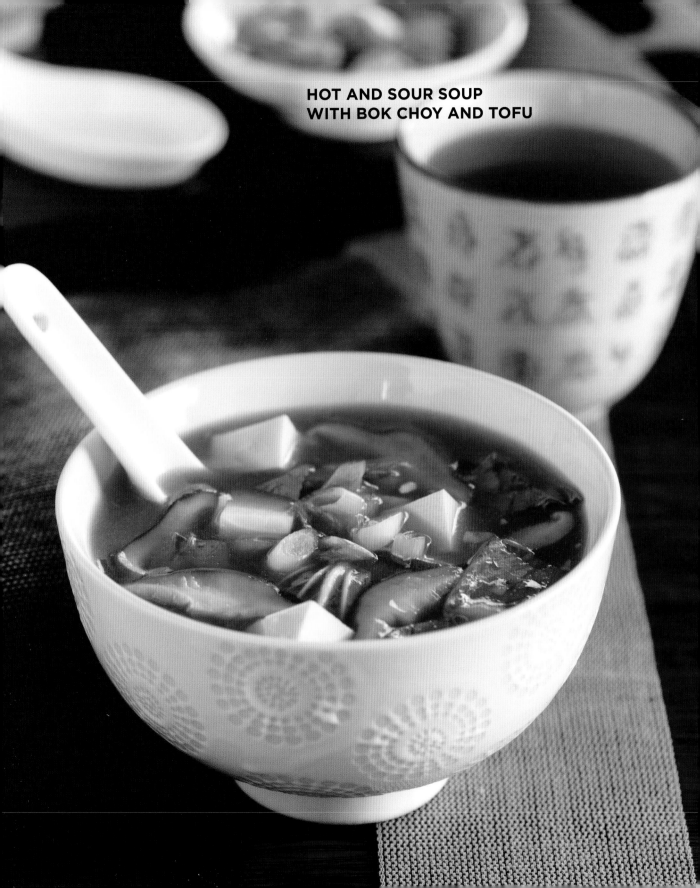

**HOT AND SOUR SOUP
WITH BOK CHOY AND TOFU**

Curried Eggplant, Squash and Chickpea Stew

 1 teaspoon olive oil

 ½ cup diced red bell pepper

 ¼ cup diced onion

1¼ teaspoons curry powder

 1 clove garlic, minced

 ½ teaspoon salt

1¼ cups cubed peeled eggplant

 ¾ cup cubed peeled acorn or butternut squash

 ⅔ cup rinsed and drained canned chickpeas

 ½ cup vegetable broth or water

 3 tablespoons dry white wine

    Hot pepper sauce

    Plain yogurt (optional)

    Chopped fresh parsley (optional)

1. Heat oil in medium saucepan over medium heat. Add bell pepper and onion; cook and stir 5 minutes. Add curry powder, garlic and salt; cook and stir 1 minute.

2. Stir in eggplant, squash, chickpeas, broth and wine; bring to a boil. Reduce heat to low; cover and simmer 20 to 25 minutes or just until squash and eggplant are tender.

3. Season to taste with hot pepper sauce. Serve with yogurt and parsley, if desired.

Makes 2 servings

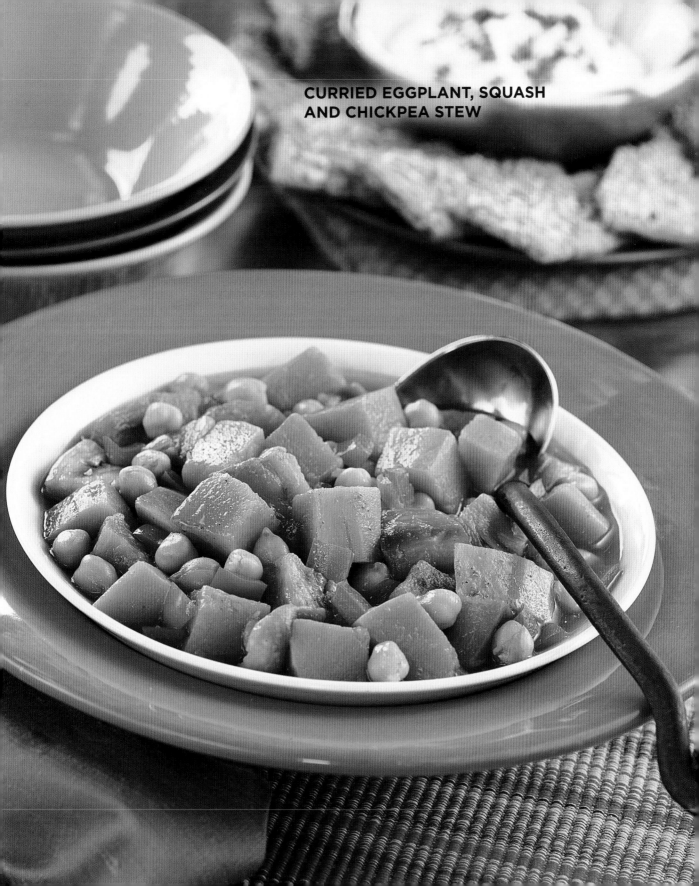

Two-Cheese Potato and Cauliflower Soup

1 tablespoon butter

1 cup chopped onion

2 cloves garlic, minced

5 cups whole milk

1 pound Yukon Gold potatoes, diced

1 pound cauliflower florets

1½ teaspoons salt

⅛ teaspoon ground red pepper

1½ cups (6 ounces) shredded sharp Cheddar cheese

⅓ cup crumbled blue cheese

1. Melt butter in large saucepan over medium-high heat. Add onion; cook and stir 4 minutes or until translucent. Add garlic; cook and stir 15 seconds.

2. Stir in milk, potatoes, cauliflower, salt and red pepper; bring to a boil. Reduce heat to low; cover and simmer 15 minutes or until potatoes are tender. Cool slightly.

3. Working in batches, blend soup in blender or food processor until smooth. Return soup to saucepan. (Or use hand-held immersion blender.) Cook and stir over medium heat just until heated through. Remove from heat; stir in Cheddar and blue cheese until melted.

Makes 4 to 6 servings

Tip: One pound of trimmed cauliflower will yield about 1½ cups of florets. You can also substitute 1 pound of frozen cauliflower florets for the fresh florets.

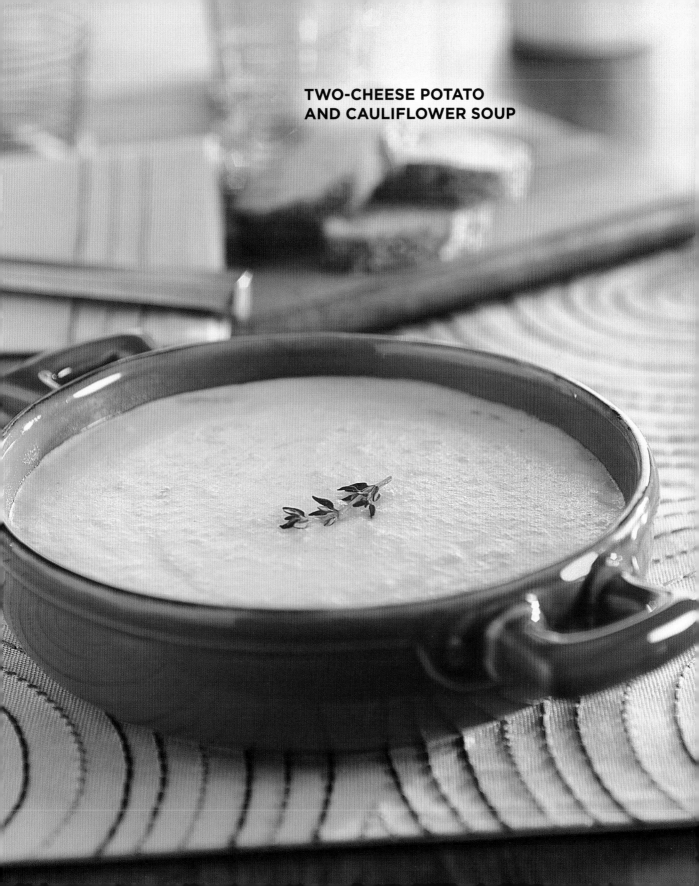

**TWO-CHEESE POTATO
AND CAULIFLOWER SOUP**

Mushroom Barley Stew

1 tablespoon olive oil

1 medium onion, finely chopped

1 cup chopped carrots (about 2 carrots)

1 clove garlic, minced

5 cups reduced-sodium vegetable broth

1 cup pearl barley

1 cup chopped dried mushrooms

1 teaspoon salt

½ teaspoon dried thyme

½ teaspoon black pepper

Slow Cooker Directions

1. Heat oil in medium skillet over medium-high heat. Add onion, carrots and garlic; cook and stir 5 minutes or until tender. Transfer to slow cooker.

2. Add broth, barley, mushrooms, salt, thyme and pepper to slow cooker; mix well.

3. Cover; cook on LOW 6 to 7 hours.

Makes 4 to 6 servings

Variation: To turn this thick, robust stew into a soup, add 2 to 3 additional cups of broth. Cook the same length of time.

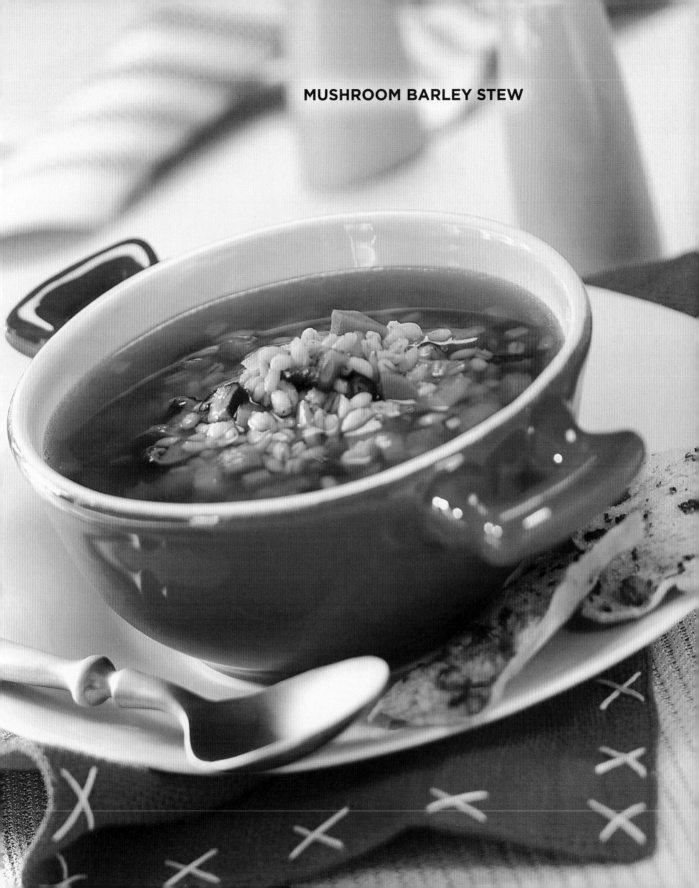

MUSHROOM BARLEY STEW

Roasted Butternut Squash Soup

1 butternut squash (about 1½ pounds)

2 tablespoons olive oil, divided

⅔ cup chopped onion

2½ cups vegetable broth

1 Granny Smith apple, peeled and cubed

½ teaspoon salt

¼ teaspoon ground cinnamon

⅛ teaspoon ground nutmeg

⅛ teaspoon black pepper

2 tablespoons half-and-half

Toasted sunflower seeds or pumpkin seeds (optional)

1. Preheat oven to 400°F. Line baking sheet with foil.

2. Peel squash; remove and discard seeds. Cut squash into 2-inch pieces; place on prepared baking sheet. Drizzle with 1 tablespoon oil; toss to coat. Spread squash in single layer. Roast 12 minutes or until almost tender.

3. Meanwhile, heat remaining 1 tablespoon oil in large saucepan over medium heat. Add onion; cook and stir about 8 minutes or until softened and lightly browned. Add broth, apple and salt; bring to a boil over high heat. Reduce heat to low; cover and simmer 10 minutes.

4. Add squash; cover and simmer 5 minutes or until tender. Working in batches, blend soup in blender or food processor until smooth. Return soup to saucepan. (Or use hand-held immersion blender.) Stir in cinnamon, nutmeg and pepper; cook, uncovered, over low heat 3 minutes. Stir in half-and-half. Serve immediately. Garnish with sunflower seeds.

Makes 4 servings

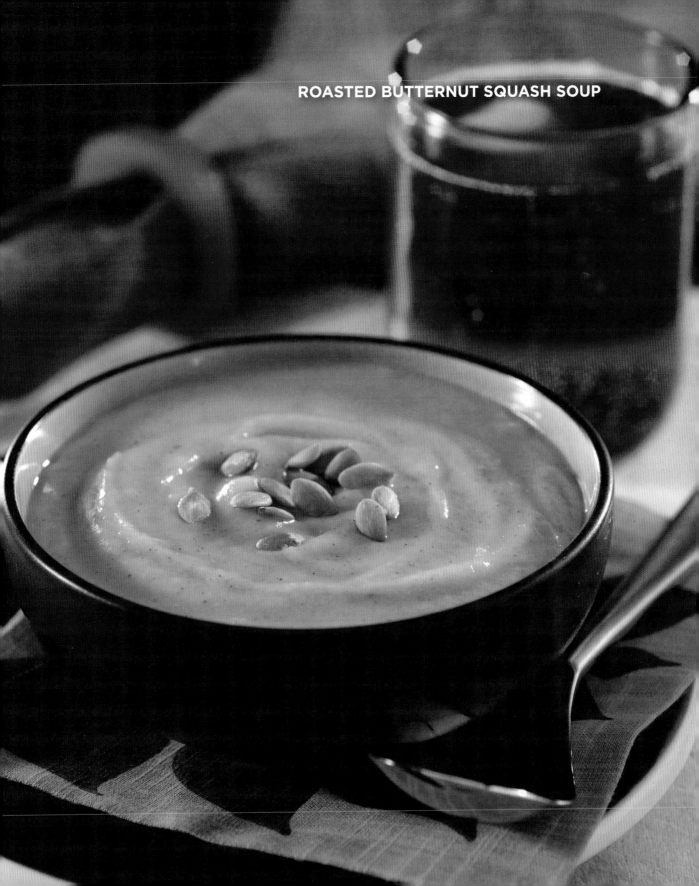

Zesty Vegetarian Chili

1 tablespoon canola or vegetable oil

1 large red bell pepper, coarsely chopped

2 medium zucchini or yellow squash (or 1 of each), cut into ½-inch pieces

4 cloves garlic, minced

1 can (about 14 ounces) fire-roasted diced tomatoes

¾ cup chunky salsa

2 teaspoons chili powder

1 teaspoon dried oregano

1 can (about 15 ounces) red kidney beans, rinsed and drained

10 ounces extra firm tofu, well drained and cut into ½-inch cubes

Chopped fresh cilantro (optional)

1. Heat oil in large saucepan over medium heat. Add bell pepper; cook and stir 4 minutes. Add zucchini and garlic; cook and stir 3 minutes.

2. Stir in tomatoes, salsa, chili powder and oregano; bring to a boil over high heat. Reduce heat to low; cover and simmer 15 minutes or until vegetables are tender.

3. Stir in beans; simmer, uncovered, 2 minutes or until heated through. Stir in tofu; remove from heat. Garnish with cilantro.

Makes 4 servings

Note: Tofu is commonly available in three forms: soft, firm and extra firm. Extra firm holds its shape well when cooked in soups and stews. Cover any leftover tofu with water and store in the refrigerator.

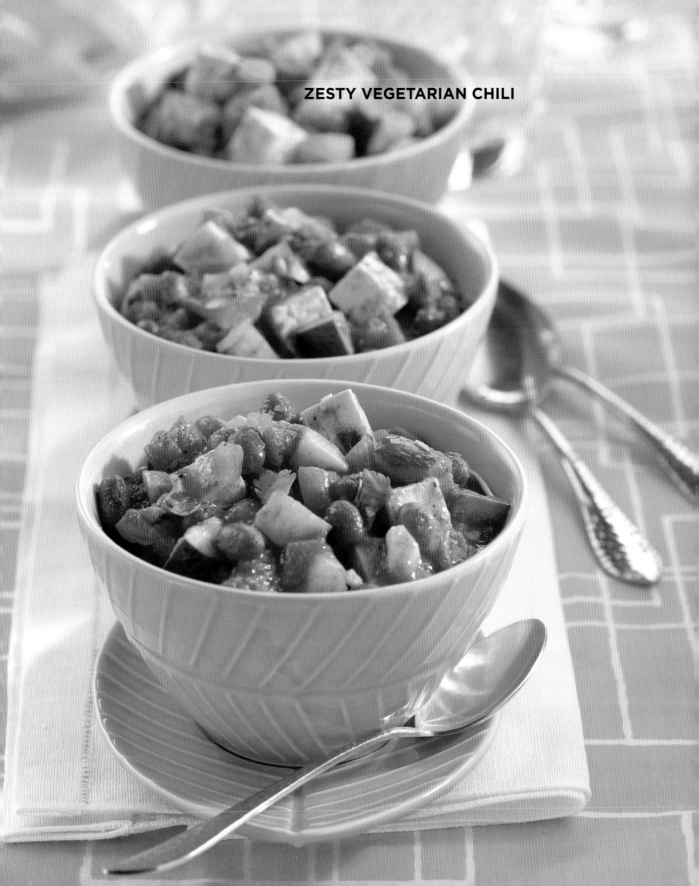

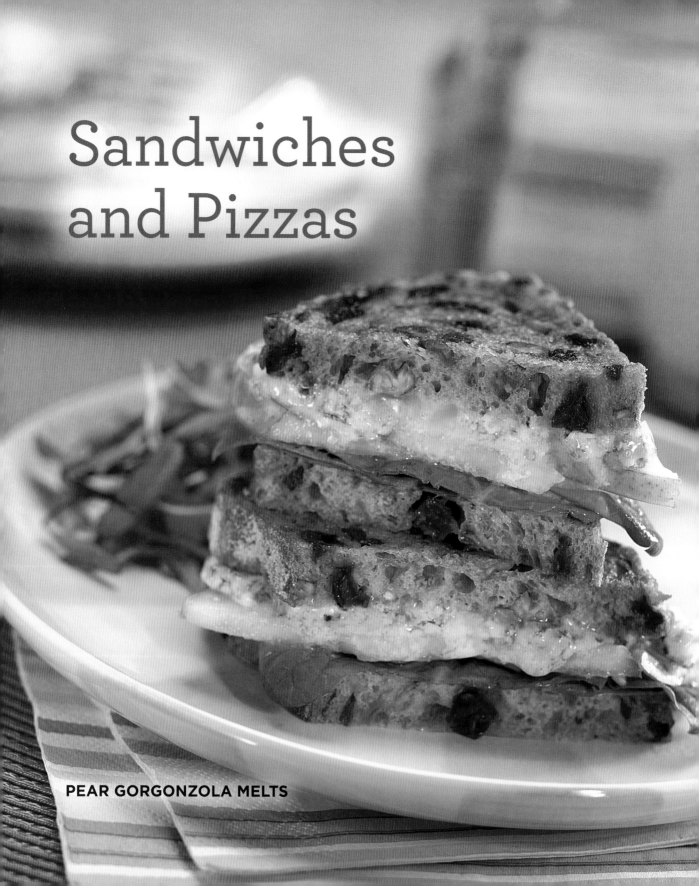

Sandwiches
and Pizzas

PEAR GORGONZOLA MELTS

Pear Gorgonzola Melts

4 ounces creamy Gorgonzola cheese (do not use crumbled blue cheese)

8 slices walnut raisin bread

2 pears, cored and sliced

½ cup fresh spinach leaves

Butter, melted

1. Spread cheese evenly on four bread slices; layer with pears and spinach. Top with remaining bread slices. Brush outsides of sandwiches with butter.

2. Heat large nonstick skillet over medium heat. Add sandwiches; cook 4 minutes per side or until cheese is melted and sandwiches are golden brown.

Makes 4 sandwiches

Spinach and Roasted Pepper Panini

1 loaf (12 ounces) focaccia

1½ cups spinach leaves (about 12 leaves)

1 jar (about 7 ounces) roasted red peppers, drained

4 ounces fontina cheese, thinly sliced

¾ cup thinly sliced red onion

Olive oil

1. Cut focaccia in half horizontally. Layer bottom half with spinach, peppers, cheese and onion. Cover with top half of focaccia. Brush outsides of sandwich lightly with oil. Cut sandwich into four pieces.

2. Heat large nonstick skillet over medium heat. Add sandwiches; press down lightly with spatula or weigh down with plate. Cook 4 to 5 minutes per side or until cheese is melted and sandwiches are golden brown.

Makes 4 servings

South-of-the-Border Pizza

  1 prepared pizza crust (about 12 inches)
  1 cup canned kidney beans, rinsed and drained
  1 cup frozen corn, thawed
  1 tomato, chopped
  ¼ cup finely chopped fresh cilantro
  1 jalapeño pepper, finely chopped
  ¼ cup (4 ounces) shredded Monterey Jack cheese

1. Preheat oven to 450°F. Place pizza crust on baking sheet.

2. Sprinkle beans, corn, tomato, cilantro and jalapeño over crust; sprinkle with cheese.

3. Bake 8 to 10 minutes or until cheese is melted and lightly browned.

Makes 4 servings

Grilled Havarti Sandwiches

  1½ teaspoons olive oil
  ⅓ cup thinly sliced red onion
  4 slices pumpernickel bread
  6 ounces dill havarti cheese, cut into slices
  ½ cup prepared coleslaw

1. Heat oil in large skillet over medium heat. Add onion; cook and stir 5 minutes or until tender. Layer two bread slices with onion, cheese and coleslaw; top with remaining two bread slices.

2. Heat same skillet over medium heat. Add sandwiches; press down with spatula or weigh down with small plate. Cook 4 to 5 minutes per side or until cheese is melted and sandwiches are browned.

Makes 2 sandwiches

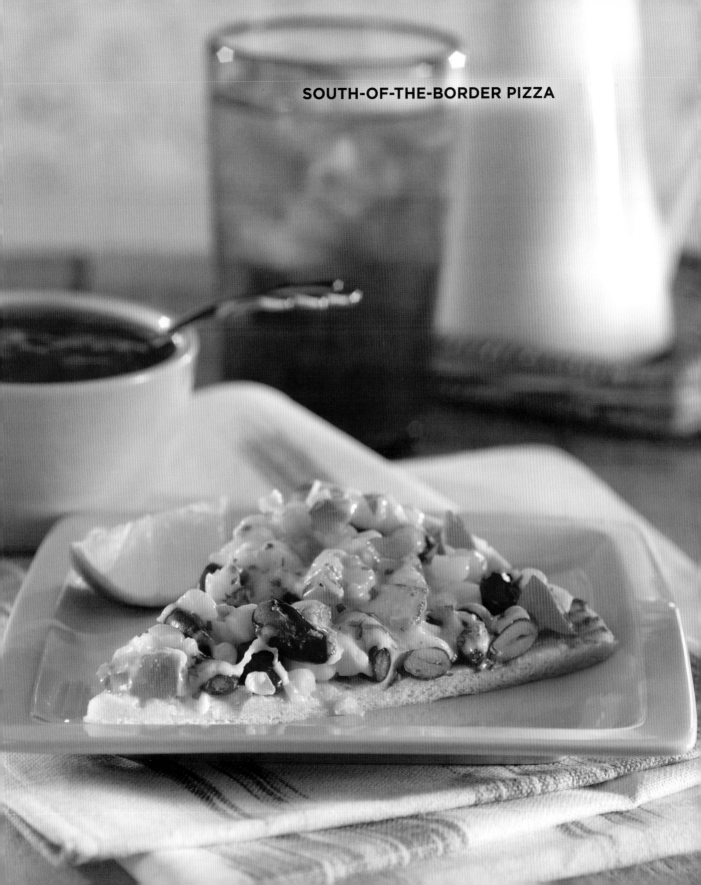

Spicy Eggplant Burgers

1 eggplant (1¼ pounds), peeled

2 egg whites

½ cup Italian-style panko bread crumbs

Nonstick cooking spray

3 tablespoons chipotle mayonnaise or regular mayonnaise

4 whole wheat hamburger buns, warmed

1½ cups loosely packed baby spinach

8 thin tomato slices

4 slices pepper jack cheese

1. Preheat oven to 375°F. Spray baking sheet with nonstick cooking spray. Cut four slices (½ inch thick) from widest part of eggplant. Beat egg whites in shallow bowl. Place panko on medium plate.

2. Dip eggplant slices in egg whites; coat with bread crumbs, pressing gently to adhere. Place on prepared baking sheet.

3. Bake 15 minutes or until golden brown. Turn and spray with cooking spray; bake 15 minutes.

4. Spread mayonnaise on bottom halves of buns; top with spinach, tomatoes and eggplant. Top with cheese and tops of buns.

Makes 4 servings

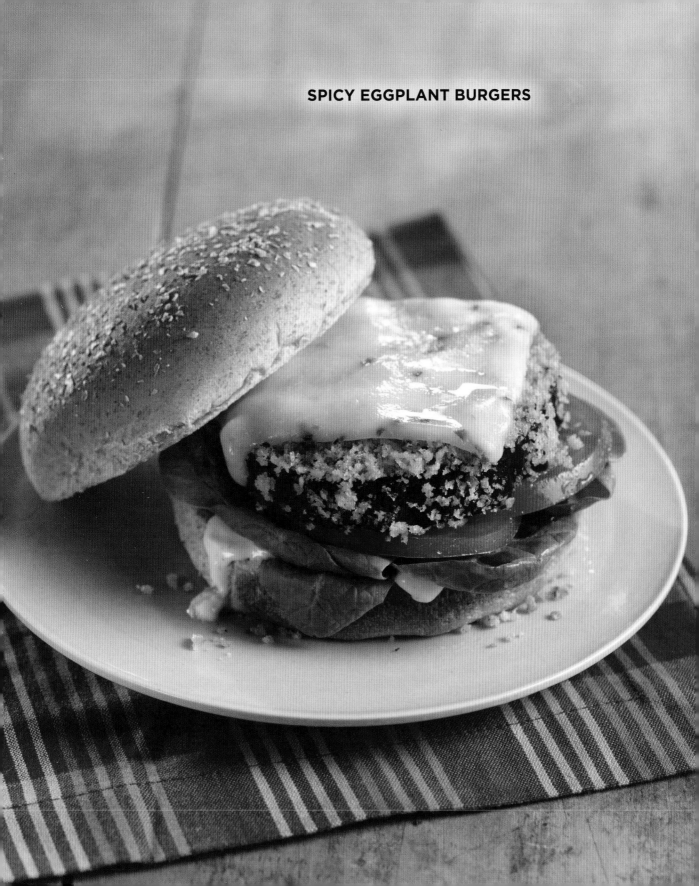

Spinach and Artichoke Pesto Pizza

1 prepared whole wheat pizza crust (about 10 ounces)

2 tablespoons prepared pesto

2 cups loosely packed baby spinach

1 can (14 ounces) artichoke hearts, rinsed, drained and chopped

1 small red bell pepper, chopped

½ cup (2 ounces) finely shredded mozzarella cheese

1. Preheat oven to 450°F. Place pizza crust on baking sheet. Spread pesto over crust; top with spinach, artichokes and bell pepper. Sprinkle with cheese.

2. Bake 10 to 12 minutes or until cheese is melted and edges of crust are brown.

Makes 4 servings

Mediterranean Pita Sandwiches

1 cup plain yogurt

1 tablespoon chopped fresh cilantro

2 cloves garlic, minced

1 teaspoon lemon juice

1 can (about 15 ounces) chickpeas, rinsed and drained

1 can (14 ounces) artichoke hearts, rinsed, drained and coarsely chopped

1½ cups thinly sliced cucumber (halved lengthwise)

½ cup *each* shredded carrot and chopped green onions

4 whole wheat pita bread rounds, cut into halves

1. Combine yogurt, cilantro, garlic and lemon juice in small bowl; mix well.

2. Combine chickpeas, artichokes, cucumber, carrot and green onions in medium bowl. Add yogurt mixture; stir gently until well blended. Divide cucumber mixture among pita halves.

Makes 4 servings

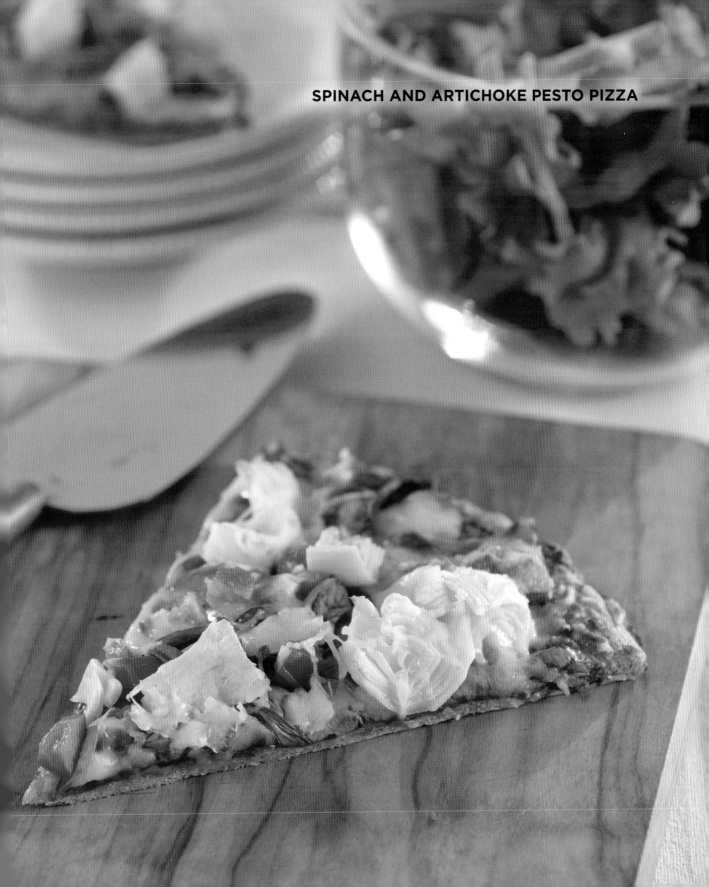

Meatless Sloppy Joes

- 1 tablespoon vegetable oil
- 2 cups thinly sliced onions
- 2 cups chopped green bell peppers
- 2 cloves garlic, finely chopped
- 2 tablespoons ketchup
- 1 tablespoon yellow mustard
- 1 can (about 15 ounces) kidney beans, rinsed, drained and mashed
- 1 can (8 ounces) tomato sauce
- 1 teaspoon chili powder
- Cider vinegar
- 4 sandwich rolls, split

1. Heat oil in large nonstick skillet over medium heat. Add onions, bell peppers and garlic; cook and stir 5 minutes or until vegetables are tender. Stir in ketchup and mustard.

2. Stir in beans, tomato sauce and chili powder. Reduce heat to medium-low; cook 5 minutes or until thickened, stirring frequently and adding up to $\frac{1}{3}$ cup vinegar if mixture is dry.

3. Serve bean mixture on rolls.

Makes 4 servings

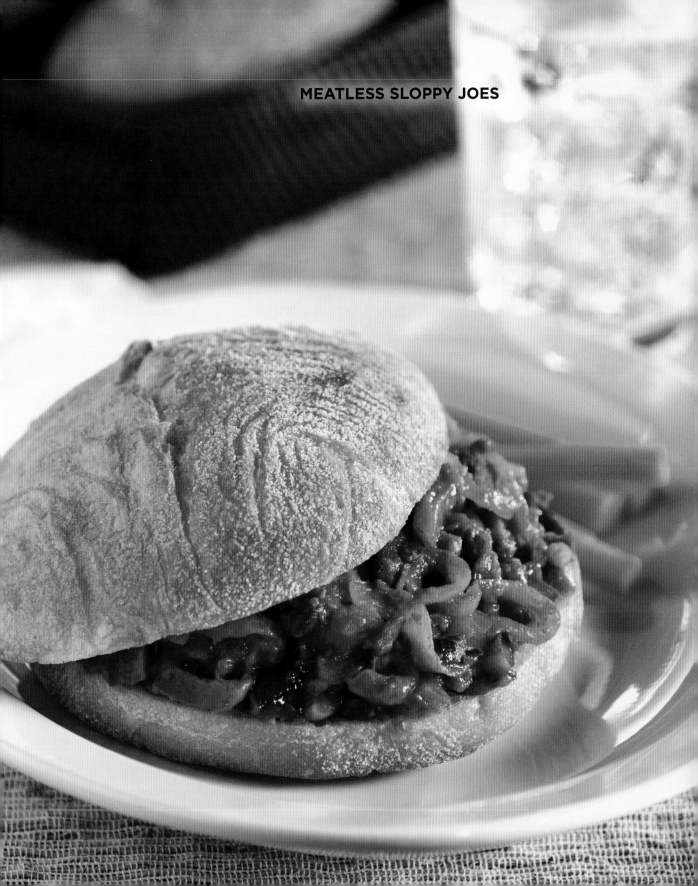

Rustic Vegetable Pizza

1 prepared whole wheat pizza crust (about 10 ounces)

2 large plum tomatoes, thinly sliced

1 tablespoon olive oil

2 small zucchini, thinly sliced

1 small eggplant, peeled and thinly sliced

⅓ cup sliced red onion

¼ teaspoon garlic salt

1 cup (4 ounces) shredded mozzarella cheese

2 tablespoons grated Romano cheese

3 tablespoons chopped fresh basil

1. Preheat oven to 450°F. Place pizza crust on baking sheet. Arrange tomatoes over crust.

2. Heat oil in large skillet over medium-high heat. Add zucchini, eggplant, onion and garlic salt; cook and stir 4 to 5 minutes or until vegetables are crisp-tender. Layer vegetables on crust over tomatoes; top with mozzarella and Romano.

3. Bake 10 to 12 minutes or until cheeses are melted and crust is golden brown. Sprinkle with basil.

Makes 6 servings

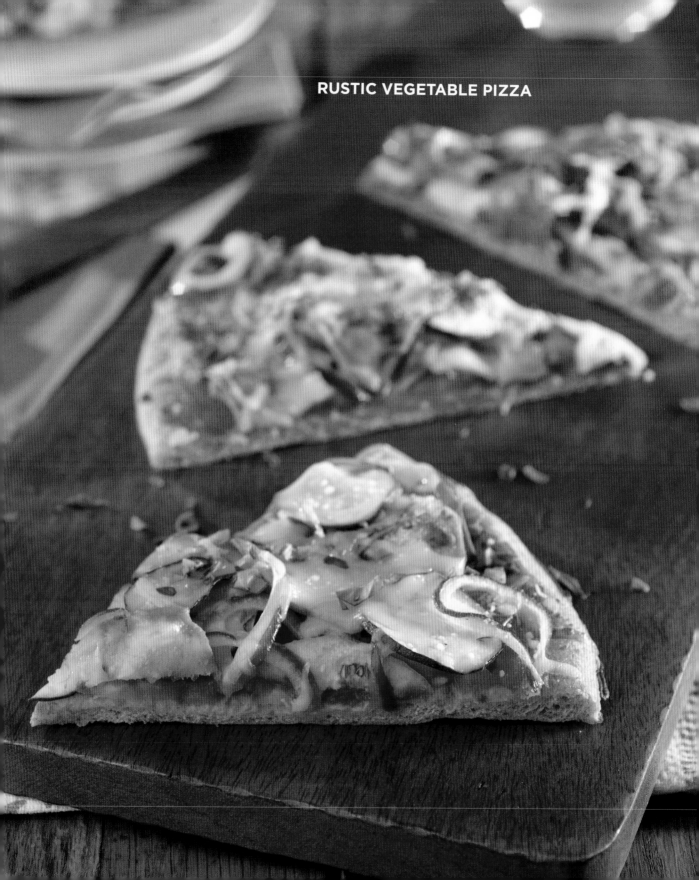

Grilled Caprese Portobello Burgers

3 ounces mozzarella cheese, diced

2 plum tomatoes, chopped

2 tablespoons balsamic vinaigrette

2 tablespoons chopped fresh basil

1 clove garlic, minced

⅛ teaspoon black pepper

4 portobello mushrooms (about 12 ounces), gills and stems removed

4 whole wheat sandwich buns, toasted

1. Prepare grill for direct cooking over medium-high heat. Oil grid.

2. Combine cheese, tomatoes, vinaigrette, basil, garlic and pepper in small bowl; mix well.

3. Grill mushroom caps, stem sides down, 5 minutes per side or until tender. Spoon one fourth of tomato mixture into each cap. Grill, covered, 3 minutes or until cheese is melted. Serve on buns.

Makes 4 servings

Note: Cooked portobello mushrooms can be frozen for several months. Store in sealed plastic containers or freezer bags.

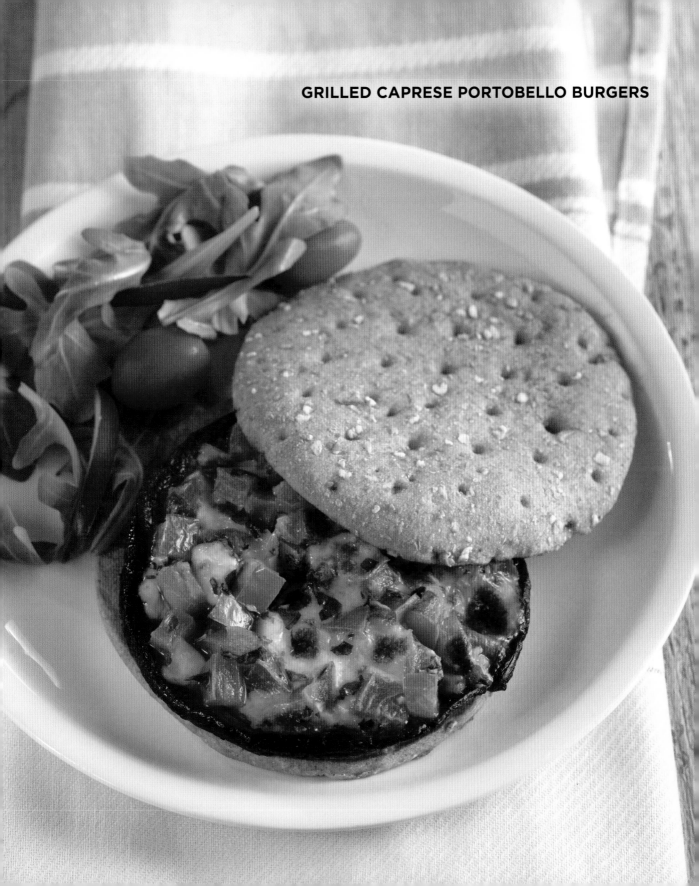

Pizza with Butternut Squash and Artichokes

2 cups diced peeled butternut squash

1 cup sliced onion

1 tablespoon extra virgin olive oil

¼ teaspoon salt

½ (9-ounce) package frozen artichoke hearts

1 prepared whole wheat pizza crust (about 10 ounces)

1 cup pasta sauce

1 cup (4 ounces) shredded mozzarella and provolone cheese blend

1. Preheat oven to 425°F. Spray baking sheet with nonstick cooking spray.

2. Combine squash and onion on prepared baking sheet. Drizzle with oil and sprinkle with salt; toss to coat. Spread vegetables in single layer. Bake 25 minutes or until squash is tender. *Increase oven temperature to 450°F.*

3. Meanwhile, prepare artichokes according to package directions. Drain and coarsely chop.

4. Place pizza crust on baking sheet or pizza pan. Spread pasta sauce over crust, leaving 1-inch border. Top with squash, onion and artichokes; sprinkle with cheese.

5. Bake 10 minutes or until cheese is melted.

Makes 4 servings

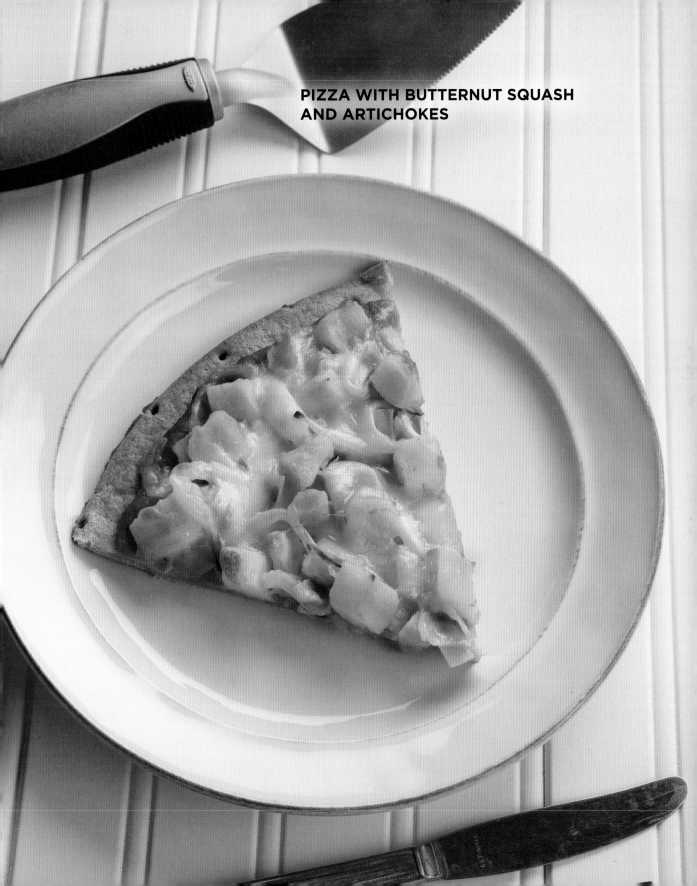

PIZZA WITH BUTTERNUT SQUASH AND ARTICHOKES

Southwestern Lentil Burgers

2 cups water

¾ cup green lentils

2 cloves garlic

1 teaspoon chili powder

1 teaspoon ground cumin

⅛ teaspoon ground red pepper

3 egg whites

⅓ cup plain dry bread crumbs

¼ cup finely chopped fresh cilantro or green onions

1 tablespoon canola oil

4 whole wheat hamburger buns, lightly toasted

⅓ cup salsa

½ ripe avocado, sliced

1. Combine water and lentils in medium saucepan; bring to a boil over high heat. Reduce heat to low; cover and simmer 20 minutes or until lentils are tender. Drain well. (Do not rinse.)

2. With motor running, drop garlic cloves through feed tube of food processor; process until minced. Add 1¼ cups cooked lentils, chili powder, cumin and red pepper; process until lentils are minced.

3. Place remaining lentils in large bowl. Add egg whites, bread crumbs, cilantro and minced lentil mixture; mix well. Shape into four patties about 4 inches in diameter. Cover and refrigerate at least 30 minutes or up to 2 hours.

4. Heat oil in large nonstick skillet over medium heat. Cook patties 5 minutes per side or until golden brown. Serve on buns with salsa and avocado.

Makes 4 servings

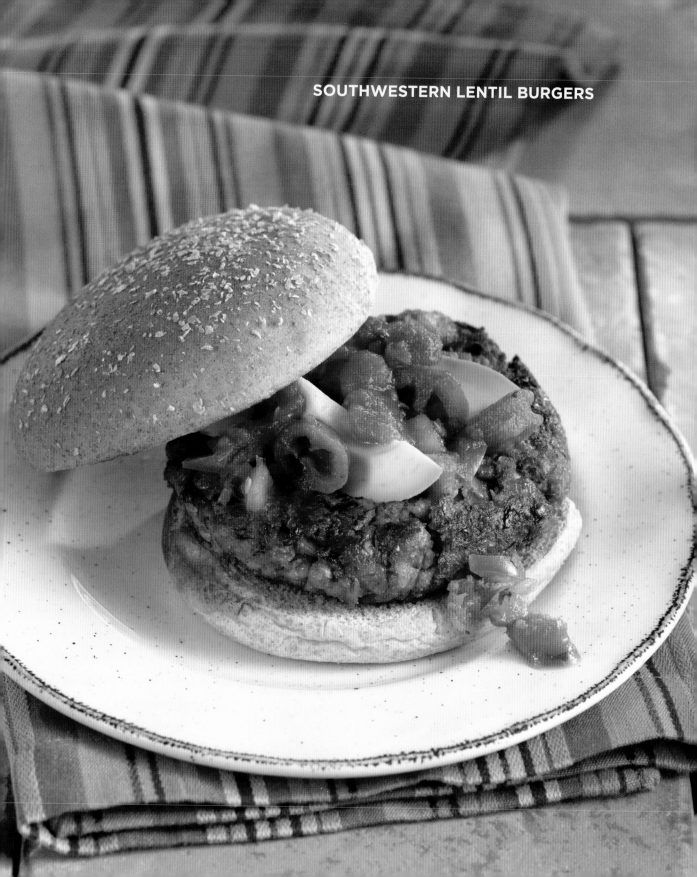

Grilled Pizza Margherita with Beer Crust

¾ cup beer

1 package (¼ ounce) active dry yeast

2 tablespoons plus 2 teaspoons extra virgin olive oil, divided

1¾ to 2½ cups all-purpose flour

1⅛ teaspoons salt, divided

1½ pints grape tomatoes, halved

1 clove garlic, minced

¼ teaspoon dried basil

⅛ teaspoon red pepper flakes

6 ounces fresh mozzarella, cut into 12 slices

10 fresh basil leaves, thinly sliced

1. Microwave beer in small microwavable bowl on HIGH 25 seconds. Stir in yeast and 2 teaspoons oil; let stand 5 minutes or until foamy. Combine 1¾ cups flour and 1 teaspoon salt in medium bowl. Add beer mixture; stir until dough pulls away from side of bowl, adding additional flour as needed. Turn out dough onto floured surface; knead 6 to 7 minutes, adding enough additional flour to make smooth and elastic dough. Divide dough in half; shape each half into a ball. Dust with flour; place in separate medium bowls. Cover and let rise in warm place about 1½ hours or until doubled in size.

2. Heat 1 tablespoon oil in medium skillet over medium-high heat. Add tomatoes garlic, basil, remaining ⅛ teaspoon salt and red pepper flakes; cook 3 to 4 minutes or until tomatoes are very soft, stirring occasionally.

3. Prepare grill for direct cooking over high heat. Oil grid.

4. Working with one ball of dough at a time, gently stretch dough into 9-inch round on lightly floured surface. Place on floured baking sheets. Brush tops of each round with half of remaining oil. Cover and let stand 10 minutes.

5. *Reduce grill to medium heat.* Carefully flip dough rounds onto grid, oiled side down. Grill, uncovered, 3 minutes or until bottoms are golden and well marked. Turn crusts; spread with tomato mixture, leaving ½-inch border.

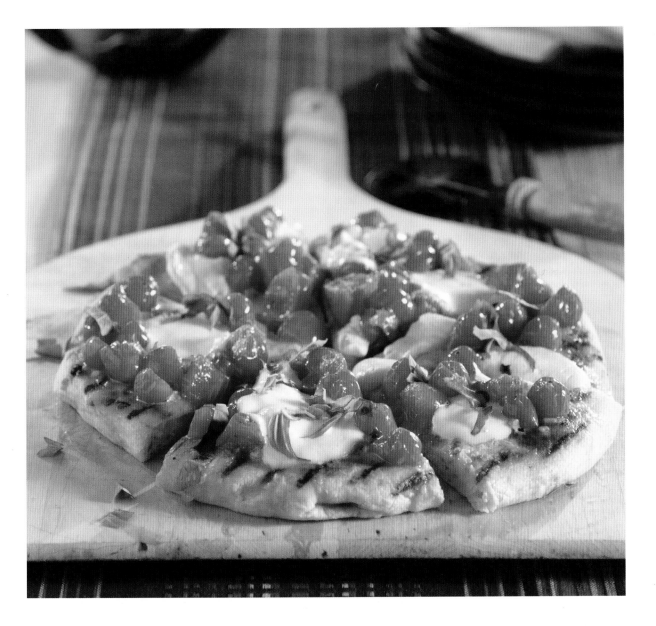

Top with cheese; cover and grill 3 minutes or until cheese begins to melt and crusts are golden brown. Remove to cutting board; sprinkle with basil.

Makes 4 servings

Portobello Provolone Panini

- 6 to 8 ounces sliced portobello mushrooms
- ⅓ cup plus 1 tablespoon olive oil, divided
- 3 tablespoons balsamic vinegar
- 1 clove garlic, minced
- ½ teaspoon salt
- ¼ teaspoon black pepper
- 1 loaf (16 ounces) ciabatta or Italian bread *or* 4 ciabatta rolls, split
- 8 ounces sliced provolone cheese
- ¼ cup chopped fresh basil
- 8 ounces plum tomatoes, thinly sliced
- 3 tablespoons whole grain Dijon mustard

1. Combine mushrooms, ⅓ cup oil, vinegar, garlic, salt and pepper in large resealable food storage bag. Seal bag; shake to coat. Let stand 15 minutes, turning frequently. (Mushrooms may be prepared up to 24 hours in advance; refrigerate and turn occasionally.)

2. Preheat indoor grill. Brush both sides of bread with remaining 1 tablespoon oil; cut bread in half lengthwise.

3. Arrange mushrooms over bottom half of bread; drizzle with some of remaining marinade. Top with cheese, basil and tomatoes. Spread mustard over remaining half of bread; place over tomatoes. Cut sandwich into four pieces.

4. Grill each sandwich 8 minutes or until cheese is melted and sandwich is golden brown. Wrap sandwiches in foil to keep warm or serve at room temperature.

Makes 4 servings

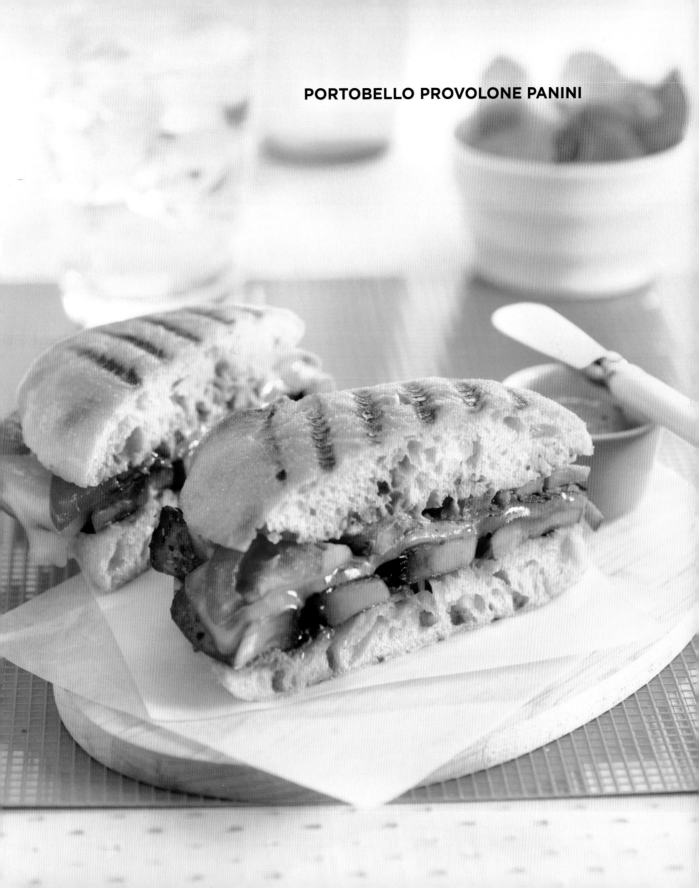

PORTOBELLO PROVOLONE PANINI

Pressed Party Sandwich

  1 (12-inch) loaf hearty peasant bread or sourdough bread

1½ cups fresh basil leaves

  6 ounces thinly sliced smoked provolone or mozzarella cheese (about 9 slices)

  3 plum tomatoes, sliced

  1 red onion, thinly sliced*

  2 roasted red bell peppers

  2 to 3 tablespoons extra virgin olive oil

  1 tablespoon balsamic vinegar

 ¼ teaspoon salt

 ¼ teaspoon black pepper

*To reduce onion's strong flavor, place onion slices in sieve or colander and rinse with cold water. Shake and pat dry.

1. Cut bread in half lengthwise. Place halves cut side up on work surface. Gently pull out some of interior, leaving at least 1½-inch bread shell.

2. Layer basil, cheese, tomatoes, onion and roasted peppers on bottom half of loaf; drizzle with oil and vinegar. Sprinkle with salt and pepper; top with remaining half of loaf.

3. Wrap sandwich tightly in plastic wrap; place on baking sheet. Top with another baking sheet. Place canned goods or heavy pots and pans on top of baking sheet. Refrigerate sandwich several hours or overnight.

4. Cut sandwich into 1-inch slices; arrange on serving platter.

Makes 12 slices

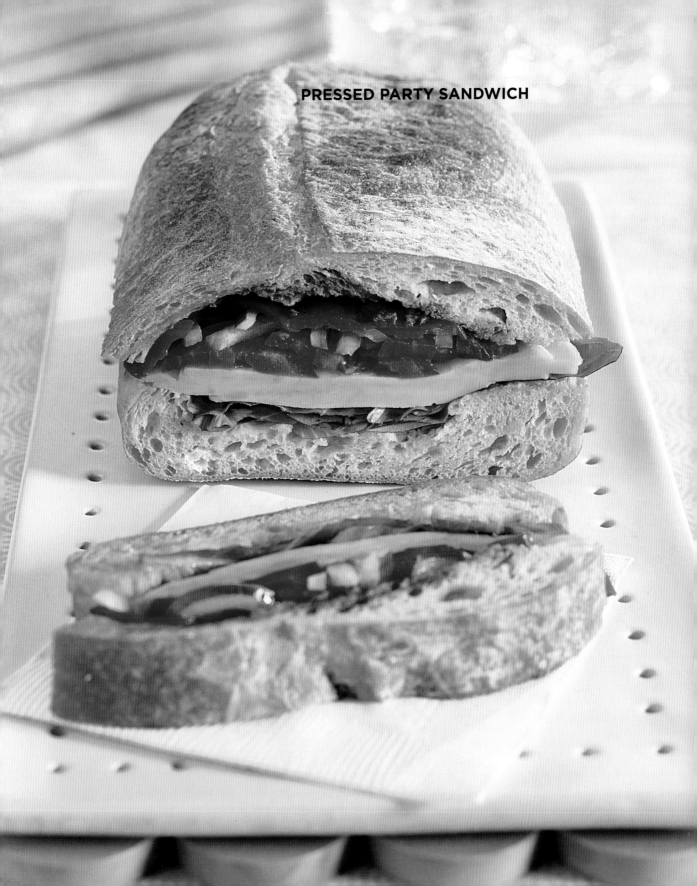

Gratin Eggs on Toast

1½ tablespoons butter

1½ tablespoons all-purpose flour

1½ cups milk

2 teaspoons Dijon mustard

¼ teaspoon salt

⅛ teaspoon black pepper

6 hard-cooked eggs, peeled

½ cup (2 ounces) shredded Cheddar cheese

6 slices toast

1. Preheat broiler. Spray 11×7-inch baking pan with nonstick cooking spray.

2. Melt butter in medium saucepan over medium-low heat. Stir in flour; cook 1 to 2 minutes, stirring constantly. Whisk in milk; bring to a boil. Cook 1 to 2 minutes or until thickened, whisking constantly. Stir in mustard, salt and pepper.

3. Chop eggs into large pieces; place in prepared pan. Pour sauce over eggs; top with cheese.

4. Broil close to heat source 1 to 2 minutes or until cheese is bubbly and begins to brown. Serve eggs and sauce over toast.

Makes 6 servings

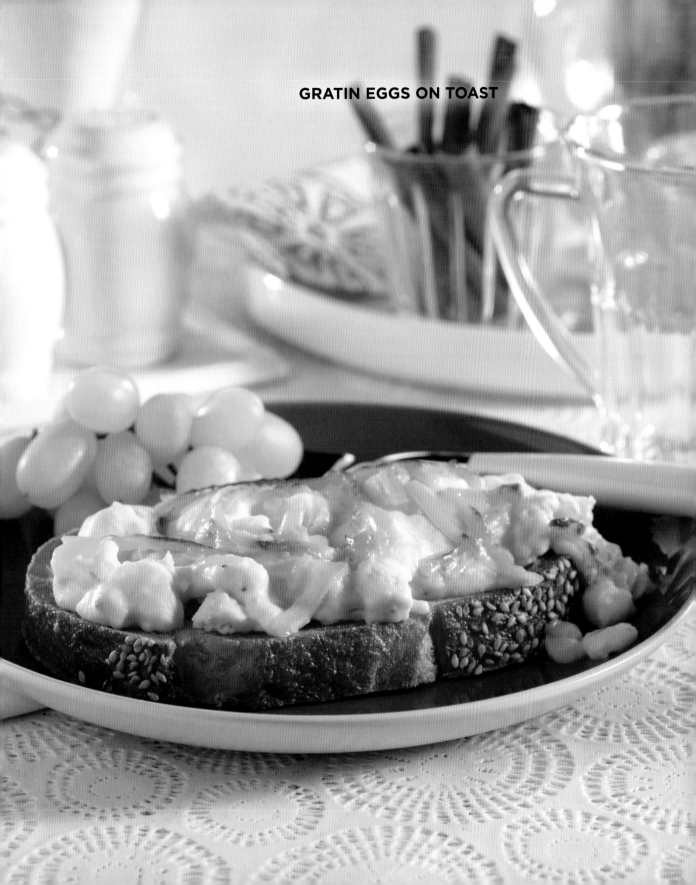

GRATIN EGGS ON TOAST

Hummus Pita Pizzas

1 can (about 15 ounces) chickpeas, rinsed and drained

3 tablespoons olive oil

2 teaspoons lemon juice

1 teaspoon minced garlic

¼ teaspoon salt

⅛ teaspoon ground red pepper

4 pita bread rounds

1 cup chopped fresh tomato

1 can (4 ounces) sliced black olives, drained

1½ cups (6 ounces) shredded mozzarella cheese

1. Preheat oven to 425°F. Combine chickpeas, oil, lemon juice, garlic, salt and red pepper in food processor or blender; process until smooth.

2. Spread hummus over pita rounds; top with tomato, olives and cheese.

3. Bake 8 to 10 minutes or until cheese is lightly browned.

Makes 4 servings

Serving Suggestion: Add a quick cucumber-yogurt salad to complete this meal. Toss chopped seeded cucumbers with plain yogurt; season with minced garlic, dried dill weed, salt and black pepper to taste.

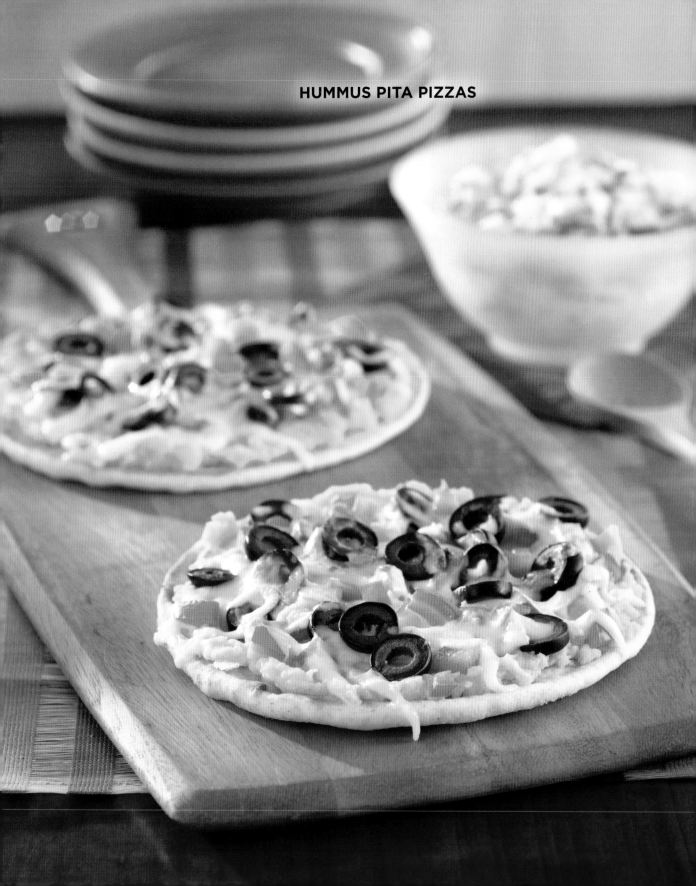

Vegan Black Bean Sliders

  6 tablespoons water

  2 tablespoons ground flax seed (see Note)

  1 can (about 15 ounces) black beans, rinsed and drained

  2 cloves garlic

  ¼ teaspoon salt

  ½ cup chopped red onion

  ½ cup chopped red bell pepper

  2 tablespoons chopped fresh parsley

  1 cup plain dry bread crumbs

  32 mini whole wheat pita bread rounds, split

     Sliced avocado and salsa (optional)

1. Combine water and flax seed in small saucepan; bring to a simmer over medium-low heat. Simmer 5 minutes or until thickened. Cool completely.

2. Preheat oven to 375°F. Spray baking sheet with nonstick cooking spray.

3. Combine beans, flax seed mixture, garlic and salt in food processor or blender; process just until smooth. Add onion, bell pepper and parsley; pulse until combined. Stir in bread crumbs.

4. Shape mixture into 32 (1-inch) patties. Place on prepared baking sheet. Spray patties with cooking spray.

5. Bake 10 minutes. Turn patties; bake 10 minutes or until lightly crisped and heated through. Serve in mini pita rounds with avocado and salsa, if desired.

Makes 32 sliders

Note: This recipe can easily be made non-vegan by substituting 2 eggs for the ground flax seed and water.

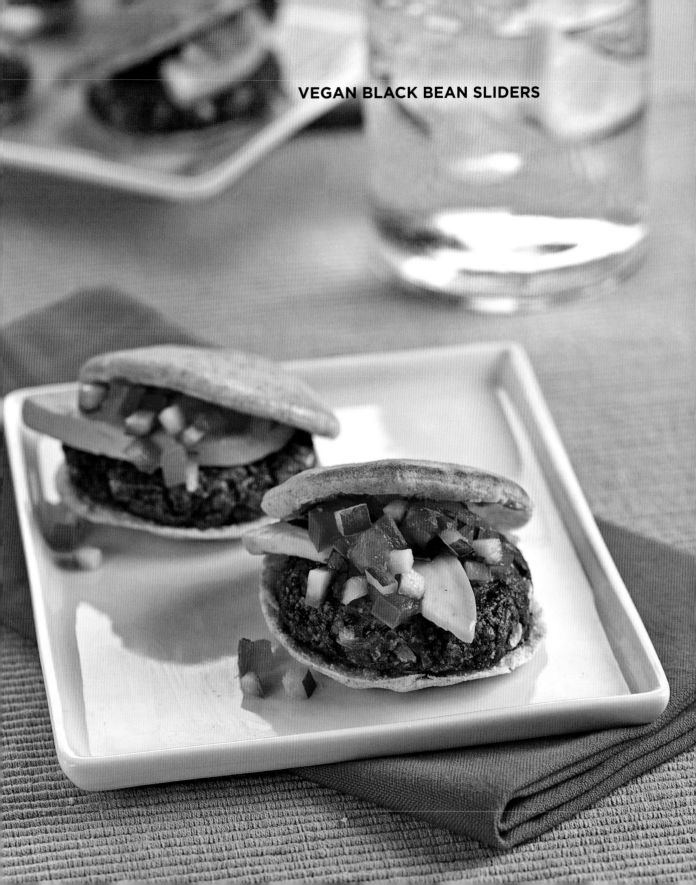

VEGAN BLACK BEAN SLIDERS

Mushroom and Goat Cheese Pizza

1 package (about 14 ounces) refrigerated pizza dough

2 tablespoons olive oil

1 red onion, thinly sliced

3 cloves garlic, minced

1 package (8 ounces) sliced button mushrooms

1 package (6 ounces) sliced cremini mushrooms

1 package (5 ounces) sliced shiitake mushrooms

Salt and black pepper

1 package (4 ounces) goat cheese, softened

2 cups (8 ounces) shredded mozzarella cheese or pizza cheese blend, divided

¾ cup sun-dried tomatoes (not packed in oil), finely chopped

1. Preheat oven to 400°F. Line baking sheet with parchment paper or spray with nonstick cooking spray. Shape dough into large rectangle on prepared baking sheet. Bake 7 minutes or until set. Cool slightly.

2. Meanwhile, heat oil in large skillet over medium-high heat. Add onion; cook and stir 2 minutes. Add garlic; cook and stir 30 seconds. Add button and cremini mushrooms; cook 5 minutes, stirring occasionally. Add shiitake mushrooms; season with salt and pepper. Cook 10 minutes or until liquid has evaporated.

3. Spread goat cheese over pizza crust; sprinkle with 1½ cups mozzarella and tomatoes. Top with mushroom mixture; sprinkle with remaining ½ cup mozzarella.

4. Bake 10 to 12 minutes or until cheese is melted and crust is golden brown. Serve immediately.

Makes 4 to 6 servings

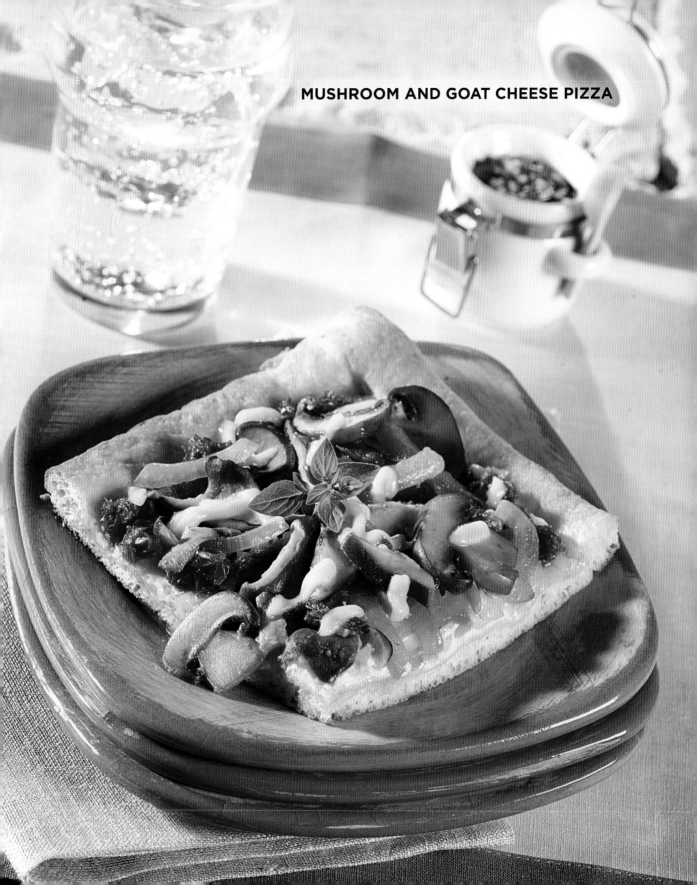

Chickpea Burgers

    1 can (15 ounces) chickpeas, rinsed and drained
    ⅓ cup chopped carrots
    ⅓ cup herbed croutons
    ¼ cup chopped fresh parsley
    ¼ cup chopped onion
    1 egg white
    1 teaspoon minced garlic
    1 teaspoon grated lemon peel
    ½ teaspoon black pepper
    ¼ teaspoon salt
    1 tablespoon olive oil
    4 whole grain hamburger buns
      Tomato slices, lettuce leaves and salsa (optional)

1. Combine chickpeas, carrots, croutons, parsley, onion, egg white, garlic, lemon peel, pepper and salt in food processor; process until blended. Shape mixture into four patties.

2. Heat oil in large nonstick skillet over medium heat. Cook patties 4 to 5 minutes per side or until golden brown.

3. Serve burgers on buns with tomato, lettuce and salsa, if desired.

Makes 4 servings

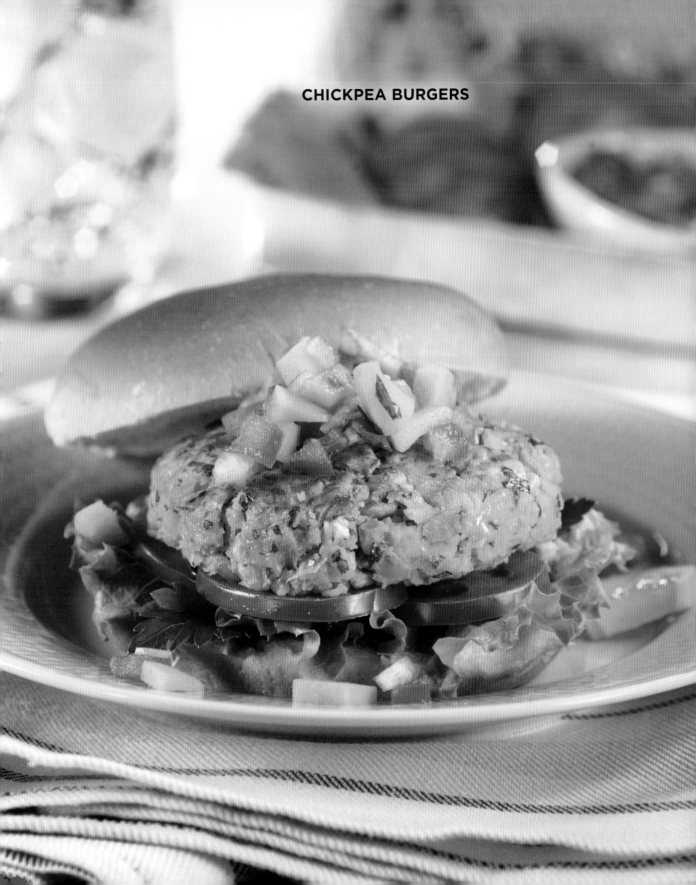

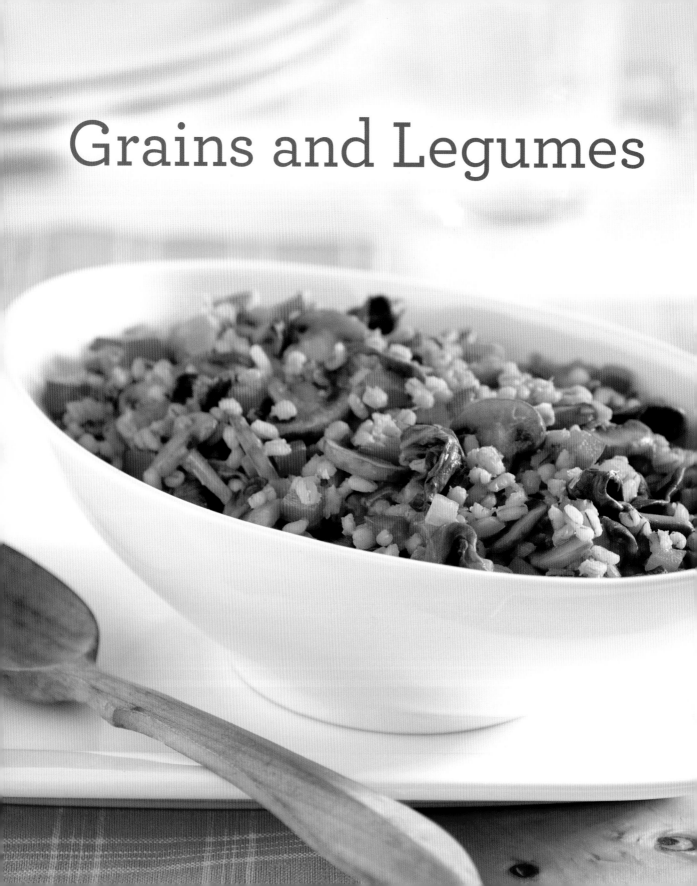

Grains and Legumes

Barley and Vegetable Risotto

4½ cups vegetable broth

1 tablespoon olive oil

1 small onion, diced

8 ounces sliced mushrooms

¾ cup pearl barley

1 large red bell pepper, diced

2 cups packed baby spinach

¼ cup grated Parmesan cheese

¼ teaspoon black pepper

1. Bring broth to a simmer in medium saucepan; keep warm over low heat.

2. Meanwhile, heat oil in large saucepan over medium heat. Add onion; cook and stir 4 minutes. Add mushrooms; cook and stir over medium-high heat 5 minutes or until mushrooms begin to brown and liquid evaporates.

3. Add barley; cook 1 minute. Add ½ cup hot broth; cook and stir until broth is almost absorbed. Continue adding broth, ½ cup at a time, stirring constantly until broth is almost absorbed before adding next ½ cup.

4. After 20 minutes of cooking, stir in bell pepper. Continue adding broth, ½ cup at a time, until barley is tender (about 30 minutes total). Add spinach; cook and stir 1 minute or just until spinach is wilted. Stir in cheese and black pepper.

Makes 4 to 6 servings

Note: Use your favorite mushrooms, such as button, crimini or shiitake, or a combination of two or more different varieties.

Heirloom Tomato Quinoa Salad

1 cup uncooked quinoa

2 cups water

¾ teaspoon salt, divided

2 tablespoons olive oil

1 tablespoon lemon juice

1 clove garlic, minced

2 cups assorted heirloom grape tomatoes (red, yellow and/or a combination)

¼ cup crumbled feta cheese

¼ cup chopped fresh basil

1. Place quinoa in fine-mesh strainer; rinse well under cold running water. Combine quinoa, 2 cups water and ½ teaspoon salt in medium saucepan; bring to a boil over high heat. Reduce heat to low; cover and simmer 15 to 18 minutes or until quinoa is tender and water is absorbed.

2. Meanwhile, whisk oil, lemon juice, garlic and remaining ¼ teaspoon salt in large bowl until well blended. Gently stir in tomatoes and quinoa. Cover and refrigerate at least 30 minutes.

3. Stir in cheese just before serving. Sprinkle with basil.

Makes 4 servings

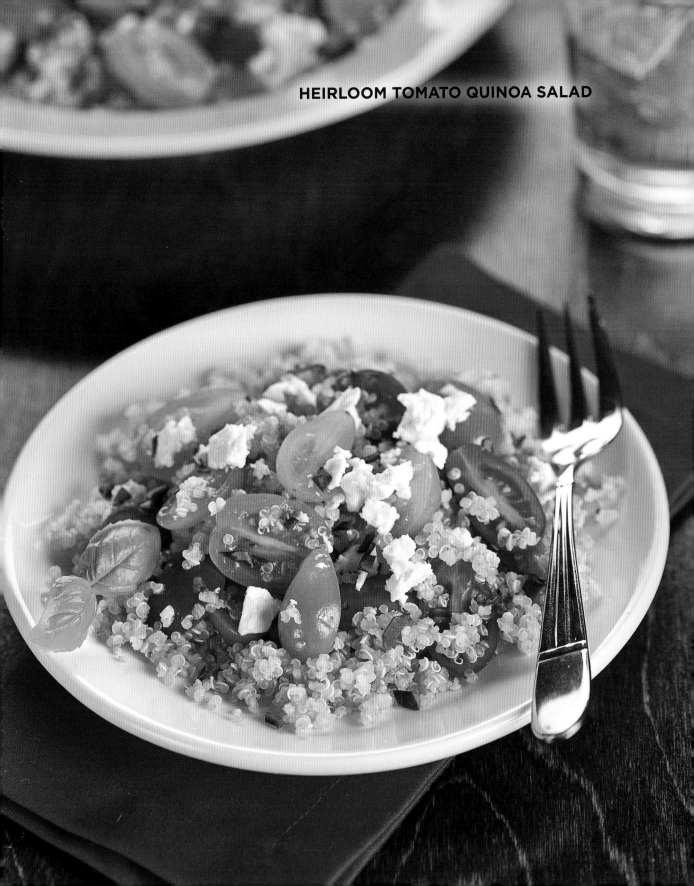

HEIRLOOM TOMATO QUINOA SALAD

Buckwheat with Zucchini and Mushrooms

1½ to 2 tablespoons olive oil

1 cup sliced mushrooms

1 medium zucchini, cut into ½-inch pieces

1 medium onion, chopped

1 clove garlic, minced

¾ cup buckwheat

½ teaspoon salt

¼ teaspoon dried thyme

⅛ teaspoon black pepper

1¼ cups vegetable broth

Lemon wedges (optional)

1. Heat oil in large nonstick skillet over medium heat. Add mushrooms, zucchini, onion and garlic; cook and stir 7 to 10 minutes or until vegetables are tender. Add buckwheat, salt, thyme and pepper; cook and stir 2 minutes.

2. Stir in broth; bring to a boil. Reduce heat to low; cover and simmer 10 to 13 minutes or until liquid is absorbed and buckwheat is tender.

3. Remove from heat; let stand, covered, 5 minutes. Serve with lemon wedges, if desired.

Makes 4 to 6 servings

Tip: Buckwheat is an excellent—and often underappreciated—option for vegetarians. It contains more protein than wheat, rice, millet or corn, and is also high in several essential amino acids. (And it contains no gluten, so it's a safe choice for those with gluten allergies or intolerance.)

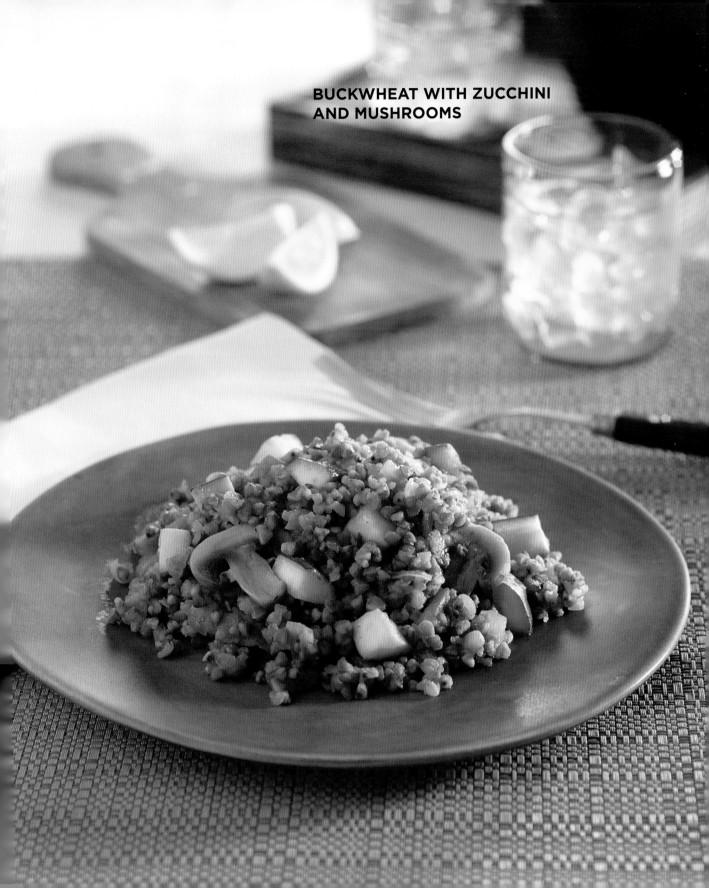

BUCKWHEAT WITH ZUCCHINI
AND MUSHROOMS

Lentil and Orzo Salad

  8 cups water

  ½ cup dried lentils, rinsed and sorted*

  4 ounces uncooked orzo pasta

1½ cups quartered cherry or grape tomatoes

  ¾ cup finely chopped celery

  ½ cup chopped red onion

  2 ounces pitted olives (about 16 olives), coarsely chopped

  3 to 4 tablespoons cider vinegar

  2 tablespoons olive oil

  1 tablespoon dried basil

  1 clove garlic, minced

  ¼ teaspoon salt

  ⅛ teaspoon red pepper flakes

  1 package (4 ounces) crumbled feta cheese with sun-dried tomatoes and basil

Packages of dried lentils may contain dirt and tiny stones. Thoroughly rinse lentils, then sort through them and discard any unusual-looking pieces.

1. Bring water to boil in large saucepan or Dutch oven over high heat. Add lentils; cook 12 minutes.

2. Add orzo; cook 10 minutes or just until tender. Drain and rinse under cold water to cool completely. Drain well.

3. Meanwhile, combine tomatoes, celery, onion, olives, vinegar, oil, basil, garlic, salt and red pepper flakes in large bowl; mix well.

4. Add lentil mixture to tomato mixture; toss gently. Stir in cheese. Let stand 15 minutes before serving.

Makes 4 servings

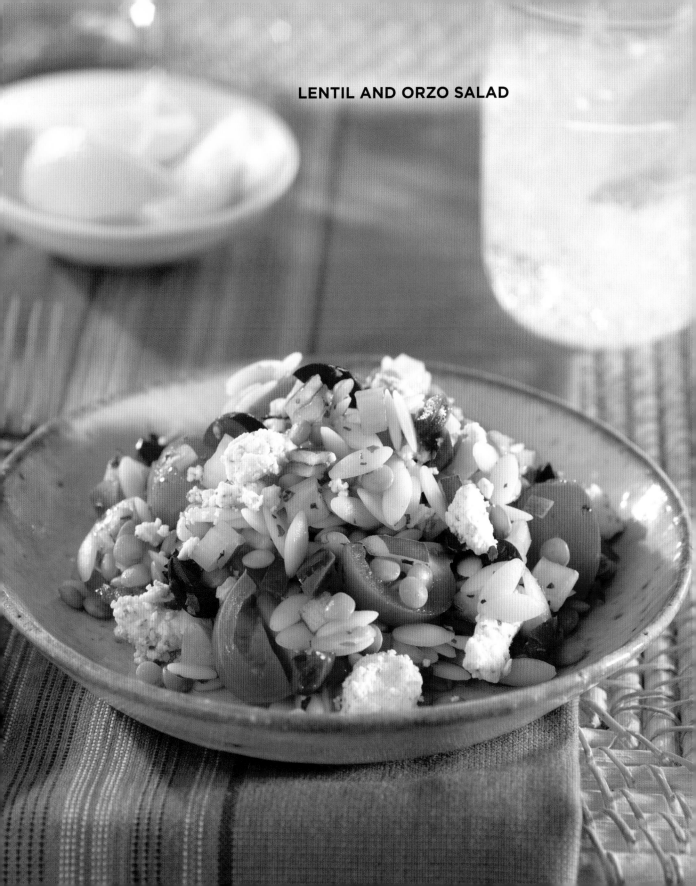

LENTIL AND ORZO SALAD

Wheat Berry Apple Salad

1 cup uncooked wheat berries (whole wheat kernels)

½ teaspoon salt

2 apples (1 red and 1 green)

½ cup dried cranberries

⅓ cup chopped walnuts

1 stalk celery, chopped

Grated peel and juice of 1 medium orange

2 tablespoons rice wine vinegar

1½ tablespoons chopped fresh mint

Lettuce leaves (optional)

1. Place wheat berries and salt in large saucepan; cover with 1 inch of water.* Bring to a boil over high heat; stir. Reduce heat to low; cover and cook 45 minutes to 1 hour or until wheat berries are tender but chewy, stirring occasionally. (Add additional water if wheat berries become dry during cooking.) Drain and let cool. (Cover and refrigerate up to 4 days if not using immediately.)

2. Cut apples into bite-size pieces. Combine wheat berries, apples, cranberries, walnuts, celery, orange peel, orange juice, vinegar and mint in large bowl; mix well. Cover and refrigerate at least 1 hour before serving. Serve on lettuce leaves, if desired.

To cut cooking time by 20 to 30 minutes, wheat berries may be soaked in water overnight. Drain and cover with 1 inch of fresh water before cooking.

Makes about 6 servings

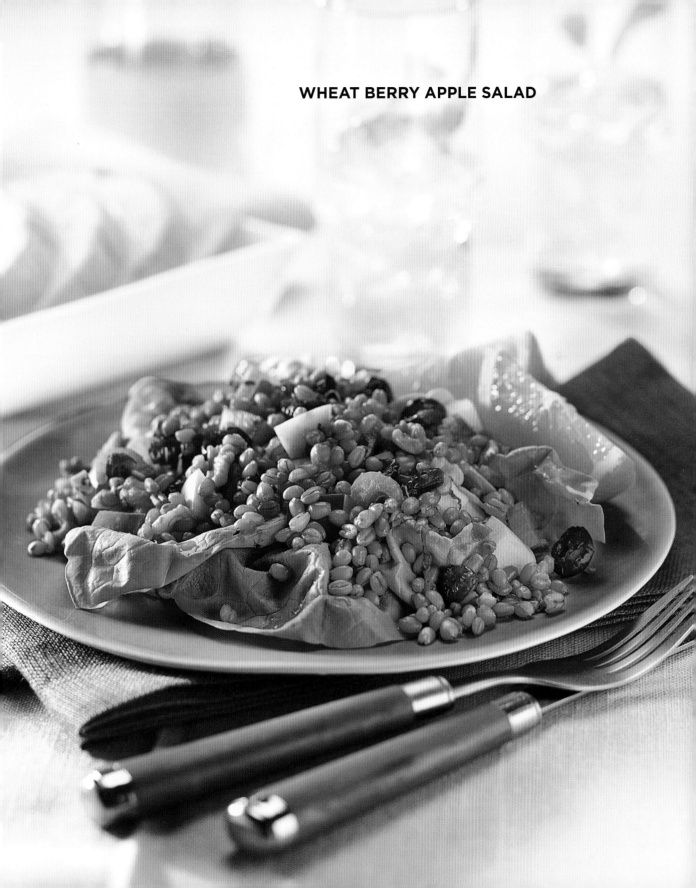

WHEAT BERRY APPLE SALAD

Polenta Lasagna

4¼ cups water, divided

1½ cups yellow cornmeal

4 teaspoons finely chopped fresh marjoram

2 medium red bell peppers, chopped

1 tablespoon olive oil

1 pound fresh mushrooms, sliced

1 cup chopped leeks

1 clove garlic, minced

½ cup (2 ounces) shredded mozzarella cheese

2 tablespoons chopped fresh basil

1 tablespoon chopped fresh oregano

⅛ teaspoon black pepper

4 tablespoons grated Parmesan cheese

1. Bring 4 cups water to a boil in medium saucepan over high heat. Gradually add cornmeal, stirring constantly. Reduce heat to low; stir in marjoram. Simmer 15 to 20 minutes or until polenta thickens and pulls away from side of pan. Spread in ungreased 13×9-inch baking pan. Cover and refrigerate about 1 hour or until firm.

2. Preheat oven to 350°F. Spray 11×7-inch baking dish with nonstick cooking spray. Combine bell peppers and remaining ¼ cup water in food processor or blender; process until smooth.

3. Heat oil in large skillet over medium heat. Add mushrooms, leeks and garlic; cook and stir 5 minutes or until leeks are crisp-tender. Stir in mozzarella, basil, oregano and black pepper.

4. Cut cold polenta into 12 (3½-inch) squares; arrange six squares in prepared baking dish. Top with half of bell pepper mixture, half of vegetable mixture and 2 tablespoons Parmesan. Top with remaining six squares polenta, remaining bell pepper and vegetable mixtures and 2 tablespoons Parmesan. Bake 20 minutes or until cheese is melted and polenta is golden brown.

Makes 6 servings

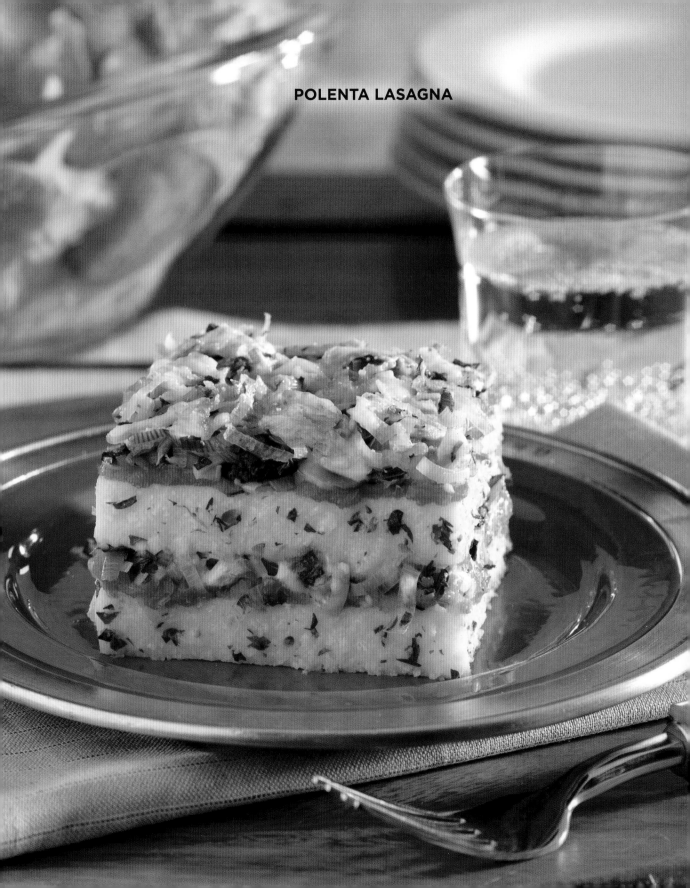

POLENTA LASAGNA

Barley and Pear-Stuffed Acorn Squash

3 small acorn or carnival squash

2 cups vegetable broth

¾ teaspoon salt, divided

1 cup quick-cooking barley

2 tablespoons butter

1 small onion, chopped

1 stalk celery, chopped

¼ teaspoon black pepper

1 large ripe pear, diced

½ cup chopped hazelnuts, toasted*

¼ cup maple syrup

½ teaspoon ground cinnamon

To toast hazelnuts, spread on baking sheet. Bake at 350°F 7 to 10 minutes or until lightly browned, stirring occasionally. Immediately remove from baking sheet; cool completely before using.

1. Preheat oven to 350°F. Pierce each squash with knife in several places. Microwave on HIGH 8 to 10 minutes or until tender, turning once. Let stand 5 minutes.

2. Cut squash in half lengthwise; scoop out and discard seeds. Arrange halves, cut sides up, in large baking dish.

3. Meanwhile, bring broth and ½ teaspoon salt to a boil in large saucepan over high heat. Stir in barley. Reduce heat to low; cover and simmer 12 minutes or until tender. (Do not drain.)

4. Melt butter in large skillet over medium heat. Add onion, celery, remaining ¼ teaspoon salt and pepper; cook and stir 5 minutes. Add pear; cook 5 minutes. Stir in barley, hazelnuts, maple syrup and cinnamon. Spoon mixture into squash halves; cover with foil.

5. Bake 15 to 20 minutes or until heated through.

Makes 6 servings

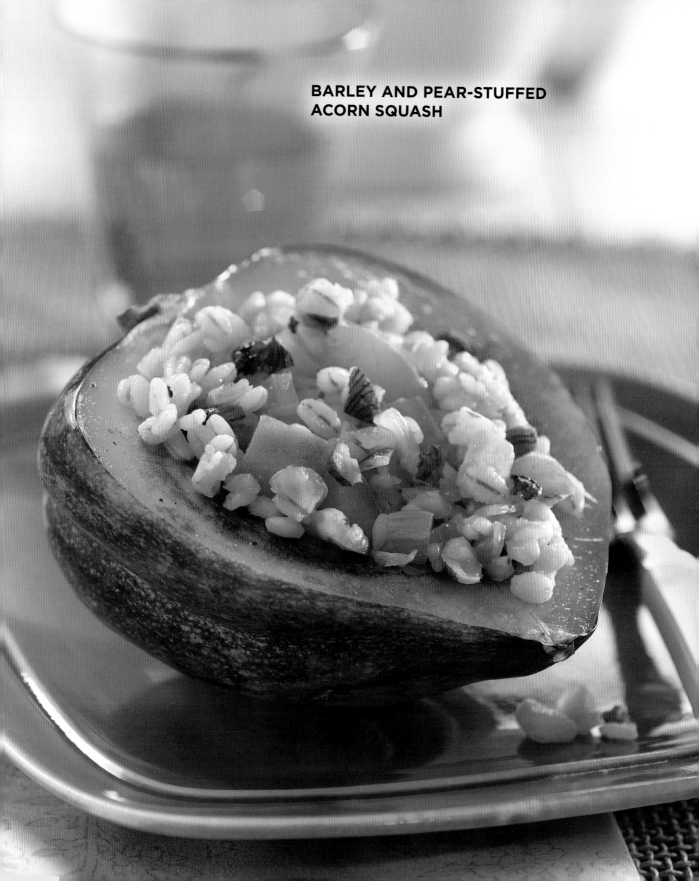

BARLEY AND PEAR-STUFFED ACORN SQUASH

Quinoa and Roasted Corn

1 cup uncooked quinoa

2 cups water

½ teaspoon salt

4 ears corn *or* 2 cups frozen corn

¼ cup plus 1 tablespoon vegetable oil, divided

1 cup chopped green onions, divided

1 teaspoon coarse salt

1 cup quartered grape tomatoes or chopped plum tomatoes, drained*

1 cup black beans, rinsed and drained

Juice of 1 lime (about 2 tablespoons)

¼ teaspoon grated lime peel

¼ teaspoon sugar

¼ teaspoon ground cumin

¼ teaspoon black pepper

Place tomatoes in fine-mesh strainer and place over bowl; let stand 10 to 15 minutes.

1. Place quinoa in fine-mesh strainer; rinse well under cold running water. Combine quinoa, 2 cups water and ½ teaspoon salt in medium saucepan; bring to a boil over high heat. Reduce heat to low; cover and simmer 15 to 18 minutes or until quinoa is tender and water is absorbed. Transfer to large bowl.

2. Meanwhile, remove husks and silk from corn; cut kernels off cobs. Heat ¼ cup oil in large skillet over medium-high heat. Add corn; cook 10 to 12 minutes or until tender and lightly browned, stirring occasionally. Stir in ⅔ cup green onions and coarse salt; cook and stir 2 minutes. Add corn mixture to quinoa. Gently stir in tomatoes and black beans.

3. Combine lime juice, lime peel, sugar, cumin and black pepper in small bowl. Whisk in remaining 1 tablespoon oil until blended. Pour over quinoa mixture; toss lightly to coat. Sprinkle with remaining ⅓ cup green onions. Serve warm or chilled.

Makes 6 to 8 servings

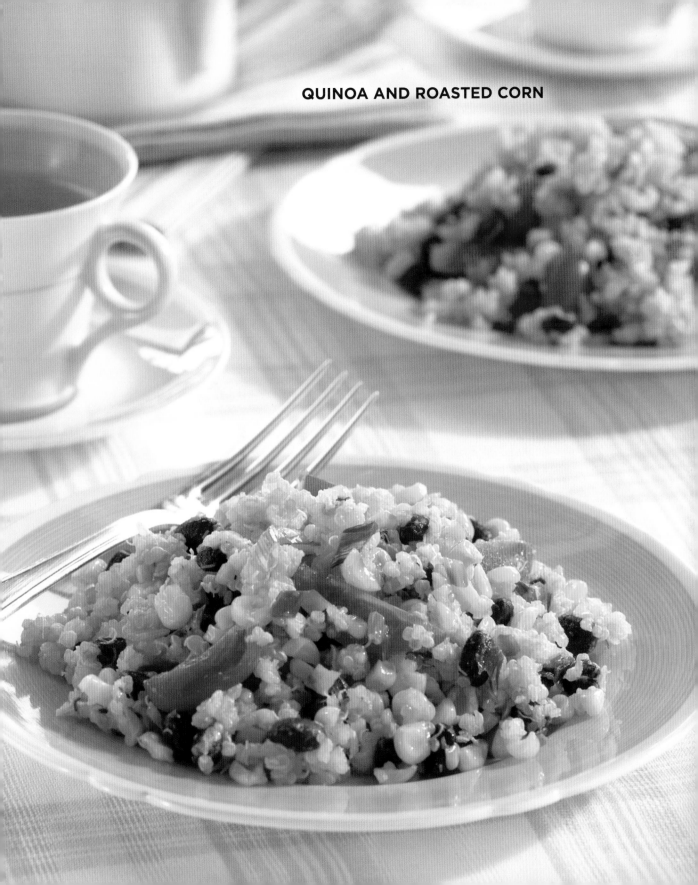

QUINOA AND ROASTED CORN

Millet Pilaf

        1 tablespoon olive oil

        ½ onion, finely chopped

        ½ red bell pepper, finely chopped

        1 carrot, finely chopped

        2 cloves garlic, minced

        1 cup uncooked millet

        3 cups water

           Grated peel and juice of 1 lemon

        ¾ teaspoon salt

        ¼ teaspoon black pepper

        2 tablespoons chopped fresh parsley (optional)

1. Heat oil in medium saucepan over medium heat. Add onion, bell pepper, carrot and garlic; cook and stir 5 minutes or until softened. Add millet; cook and stir 5 minutes or until lightly toasted.

2. Stir in water, lemon peel, lemon juice, salt and black pepper; bring to a boil. Reduce heat to low; cover and simmer 30 minutes or until water is absorbed and millet is tender. Let stand, covered, 5 minutes. Fluff with fork. Sprinkle with parsley, if desired.

Makes 6 servings

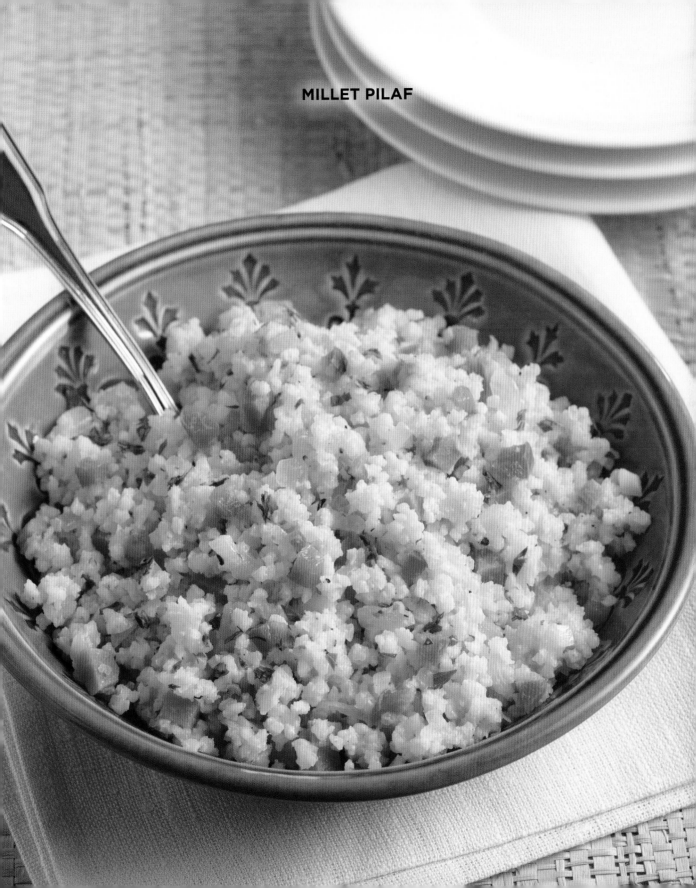

MILLET PILAF

Black Bean and Mushroom Chilaquiles

- 2 tablespoons olive oil
- 1 medium onion, chopped
- 1 medium green bell pepper, chopped
- 1 jalapeño or serrano pepper,* seeded and minced
- 2 cans (about 15 ounces each) black beans, rinsed and drained
- 1 can (about 14 ounces) diced tomatoes
- 10 ounces white mushrooms, cut into quarters
- 1½ teaspoons ground cumin
- 1½ teaspoons dried oregano
- 1 cup (4 ounces) shredded sharp Cheddar cheese, plus additional for garnish
- 6 cups tortilla chips

Jalapeño and serrano peppers can sting and irritate the skin, so wear rubber gloves when handling peppers and do not touch your eyes.

Slow Cooker Directions

1. Heat oil in medium skillet over medium heat. Add onion, bell pepper and jalapeño; cook about 4 minutes or until onion softens, stirring occasionally. Transfer to slow cooker. Add beans, tomatoes, mushrooms, cumin and oregano. Cover; cook on LOW 6 hours or on HIGH 3 hours.

2. Sprinkle 1 cup cheese over bean mixture. Cover; cook until cheese is melted. Stir to combine.

3. Coarsely crush tortilla chips. Top with black bean mixture; sprinkle with additional cheese.

Makes 6 servings

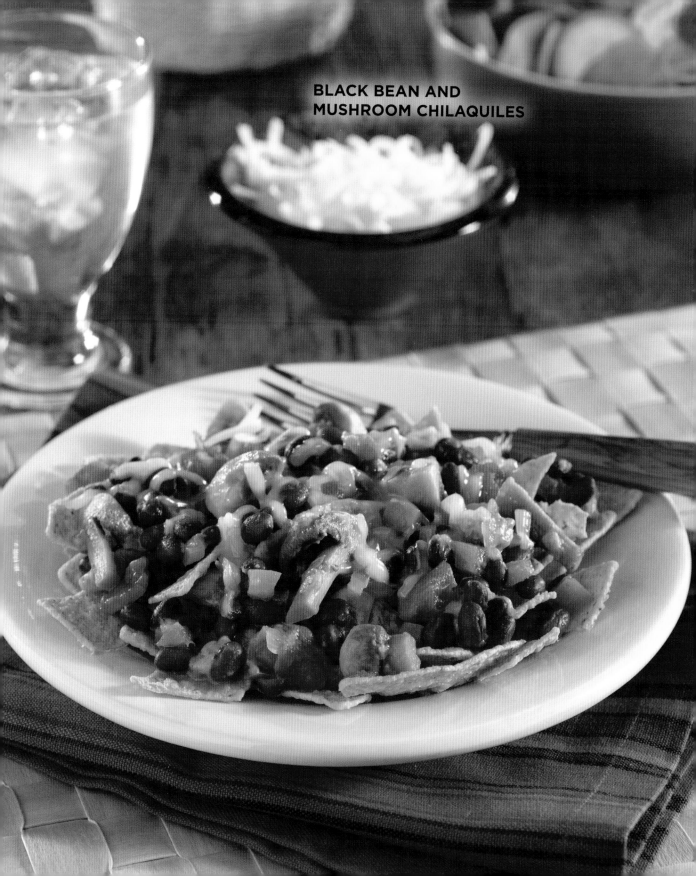

BLACK BEAN AND
MUSHROOM CHILAQUILES

Lentil Patties with Coconut-Mango Relish

1¼ cups dried lentils, rinsed and sorted

Coconut-Mango Relish (recipe follows)

1 small onion, chopped

2 cloves garlic, minced

½ teaspoon salt

½ teaspoon ground cumin

¼ teaspoon black pepper

⅛ teaspoon hot pepper sauce

1 small carrot, shredded

¼ cup all-purpose flour

1 egg

2 tablespoons chopped pitted black olives

Vegetable oil

1. Place lentils in 2-quart saucepan; cover with 2 inches of water. Bring to a boil over high heat. Reduce heat to low; cover and simmer 30 to 40 minutes or until lentils are tender. Drain and spread on paper towel-lined baking sheet. Let stand about 20 minutes or until lentils are cool and most of moisture has been absorbed. Meanwhile, prepare Coconut-Mango Relish.

2. Combine half of lentils, onion, garlic, salt, cumin, black pepper and hot pepper sauce in food processor; process just until combined (mixture will be thick). Add carrot, flour, egg and olives; pulse until well blended. Transfer to large bowl; stir in remaining half of lentils with spoon.

3. Coat bottom of large skillet with oil; heat over medium-high heat. Shape 2 rounded tablespoonfuls of lentil mixture into patty. Repeat with remaining lentil mixture. Cook patties over medium heat 6 to 7 minutes per side or until browned, adding additional oil if needed. Serve with relish.

Makes 4 to 6 servings

Coconut-Mango Relish: Combine ½ cup shredded coconut, ½ cup fresh cilantro, 2 tablespoons fresh ginger, 2 tablespoons lemon juice and 1 tablespoon water in food processor; process until finely chopped. Stir in ½ cup chopped mango.

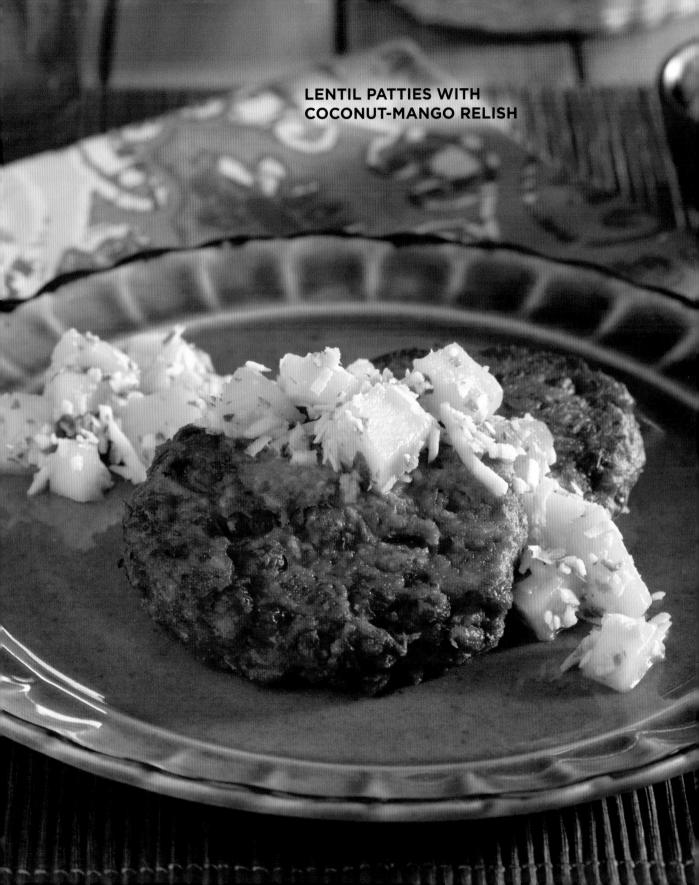

LENTIL PATTIES WITH COCONUT-MANGO RELISH

Parmesan Polenta

    4 cups vegetable broth
    1 small onion, minced
    4 cloves garlic, minced
    1 tablespoon minced fresh rosemary leaves *or* 1 teaspoon dried rosemary
    ½ teaspoon salt
  1¼ cups yellow cornmeal
    6 tablespoons grated Parmesan cheese
    1 tablespoon olive oil, divided

1. Spray 11×7-inch baking pan with nonstick cooking spray. Spray one side of 7-inch-long sheet of waxed paper with cooking spray.

2. Combine broth, onion, garlic, rosemary and salt in medium saucepan; bring to a boil over high heat. Gradually add cornmeal, stirring constantly. Reduce heat to medium; simmer 30 minutes or until mixture has consistency of thick mashed potatoes. Remove from heat; stir in cheese.

3. Spread polenta evenly in prepared pan; place waxed paper, sprayed side down, on polenta and smooth surface. (If surface is bumpy, it is more likely to stick to grill.) Cool on wire rack 15 minutes or until firm. Remove waxed paper; cut polenta into six squares and remove from pan.

4. Prepare grill for direct cooking over medium-low heat. Oil grid. Brush tops of squares with half of oil. Grill polenta, oil side down on covered grill 6 to 8 minutes or until golden brown. Brush with remaining oil; turn and grill 6 to 8 minutes or until golden brown. Serve warm.

Makes 6 servings

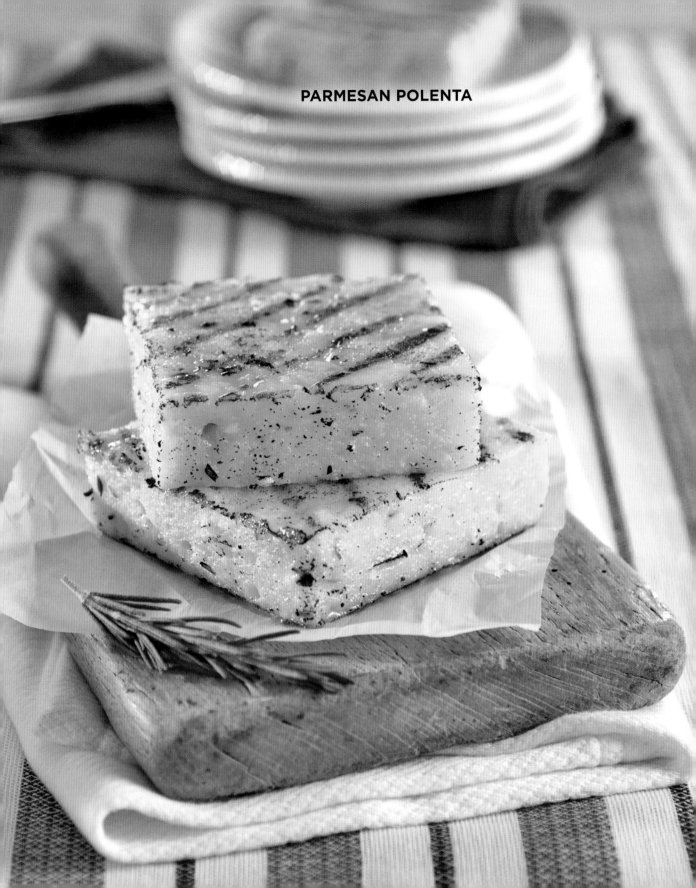

PARMESAN POLENTA

Vegetarian Paella

   1 tablespoon olive oil
   1 cup chopped onion
   2 cloves garlic, minced
   1 cup uncooked brown rice
2¼ cups vegetable broth
   1 teaspoon Italian seasoning
  ¾ teaspoon salt
  ½ teaspoon ground turmeric
  ⅛ teaspoon ground red pepper
   1 can (about 14 ounces) stewed tomatoes
   1 cup chopped red bell pepper
   1 cup coarsely chopped carrots
   1 can (14 ounces) quartered artichoke hearts, drained
   1 small zucchini, halved lengthwise and cut into ¼-inch slices
        (about 1¼ cups)
  ½ cup frozen baby peas

1. Heat oil in large nonstick skillet over medium-high heat. Add onion and garlic; cook and stir 6 to 7 minutes or until onion is translucent. Add rice; cook and stir 1 minute.

2. Add broth, Italian seasoning, salt, turmeric and ground red pepper; bring to a boil. Reduce heat to medium-low; cover and simmer 30 minutes.

3. Stir in tomatoes, bell pepper and carrots; cover and cook 10 minutes.

4. Stir in artichokes, zucchini and peas; cover and cook over low heat 10 minutes or until vegetables are crisp-tender.

Makes 6 servings

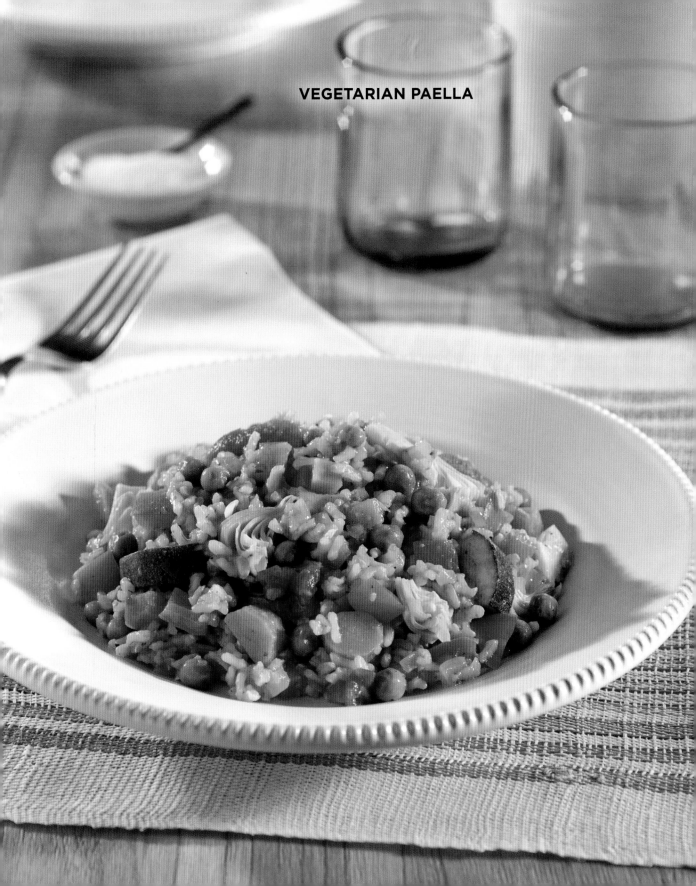

VEGETARIAN PAELLA

Grilled Fruits with Orange Couscous

1⅓ cups quick-cooking couscous

½ teaspoon ground cinnamon

½ cup orange juice

2 tablespoons vegetable oil, divided

1 tablespoon soy sauce

1 tablespoon maple syrup

⅛ teaspoon ground nutmeg

½ cup raisins

½ cup chopped walnuts or pecans

2 ripe mangoes, quartered

½ fresh pineapple, cut into ½-inch slices

1. Prepare grill for direct cooking over medium-high heat. Oil grid.

2. Prepare couscous according to package directions, adding cinnamon to water with couscous.

3. Meanwhile, whisk orange juice, 1 tablespoon oil, soy sauce and maple syrup in glass measuring cup. Combine remaining 1 tablespoon oil and nutmeg in small bowl.

4. Cool couscous 5 minutes. Stir in orange juice mixture, raisins and walnuts; mix well.

5. Place mangoes, skin side down, and pineapple on grid. Brush fruits with nutmeg mixture. Grill 5 to 7 minutes or until fruits soften, turning halfway through grilling time. Serve grilled fruits with couscous.

Makes 4 servings

Tip: To save time, purchase pineapple already trimmed and cored in the refrigerated produce section of the supermarket.

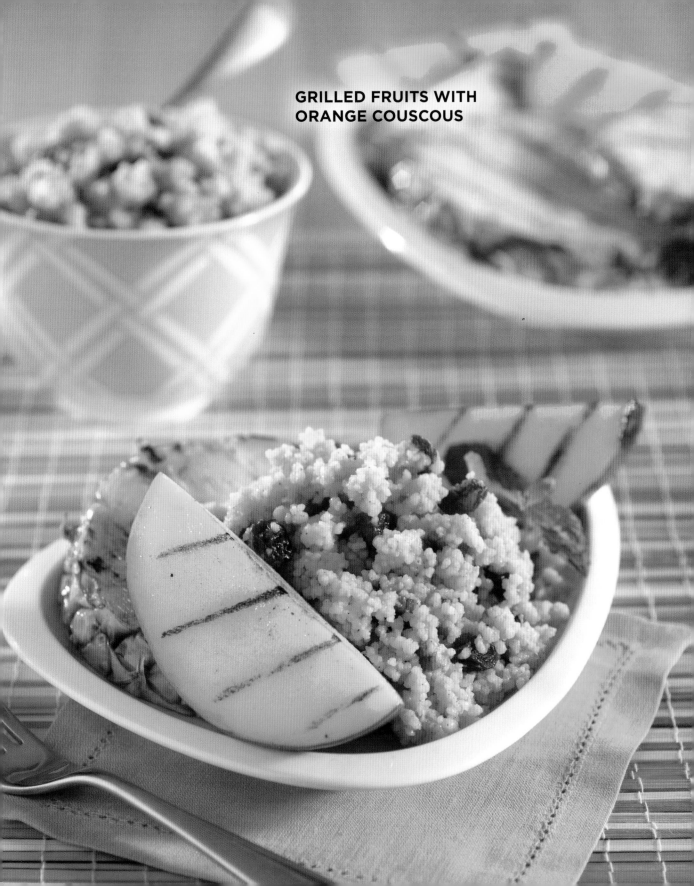

GRILLED FRUITS WITH
ORANGE COUSCOUS

Veggie "Meatballs"

½ cup water

¾ cup uncooked bulgur wheat

1 tablespoon olive oil

3 medium portobello mushrooms (10 ounces), stemmed and chopped

1 small onion, chopped

1 small zucchini (6 ounces), coarsely grated

1 teaspoon Italian seasoning

2 cloves garlic, minced

¼ cup sun-dried tomatoes (not packed in oil*), chopped

4 ounces grated Parmesan cheese

1 egg

2 cups marinara sauce, heated

*If unavailable, substitute ¼ cup sun-dried tomatoes packed in oil, well drained, patted dry and chopped.

1. Preheat oven to 375°F. Line large rimmed baking sheet with foil; spray with nonstick cooking spray.

2. Bring water to a boil in small saucepan; remove from heat. Stir in bulgur; let stand, covered, while preparing vegetables.

3. Heat oil in large skillet over medium-high heat. Add mushrooms, onion, zucchini and Italian seasoning; cook and stir about 8 minutes or until vegetables are softened. Add garlic; cook and stir 1 minute. Stir in tomatoes.

4. Transfer mushroom mixture to large bowl; let cool slightly. Add bulgur, cheese and egg; mix well. Shape into 12 balls using ¼ cup mixture for each. Place meatballs on prepared baking sheet.

5. Bake 20 minutes. Turn meatballs; bake 8 to 10 minutes or until well browned. Serve hot with marinara sauce.

Makes 4 servings

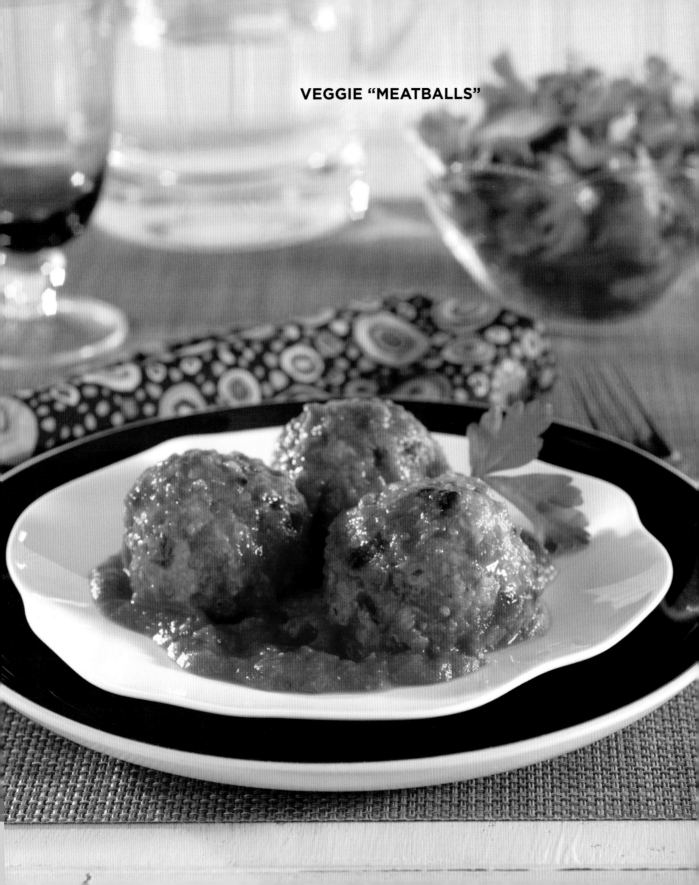
VEGGIE "MEATBALLS"

Mixed Grain Tabbouleh

3 cups vegetable broth, divided
1 cup uncooked long grain brown rice
½ cup uncooked bulgur wheat
1 cup chopped fresh tomatoes
½ cup chopped green onions
¼ cup chopped fresh mint
¼ cup chopped fresh basil
¼ cup chopped fresh oregano
3 tablespoons lemon juice
3 tablespoons olive oil
½ teaspoon salt
½ teaspoon black pepper

1. Combine 2 cups broth and brown rice in medium saucepan; bring to a boil over medium-high heat. Reduce heat to low; cover and simmer about 45 minutes or until rice is tender and broth is absorbed. Set aside to cool.

2. Combine bulgur and remaining 1 cup broth in small saucepan; bring to a boil over medium-high heat. Reduce heat to low; cover and simmer 15 minutes or until bulgur is fluffy and broth is absorbed. Cool slightly.

3. Combine tomatoes, green onions, mint, basil, oregano, lemon juice, oil, salt and pepper in large bowl; mix well. Stir in rice and bulgur. Cool to room temperature.

Makes 6 servings

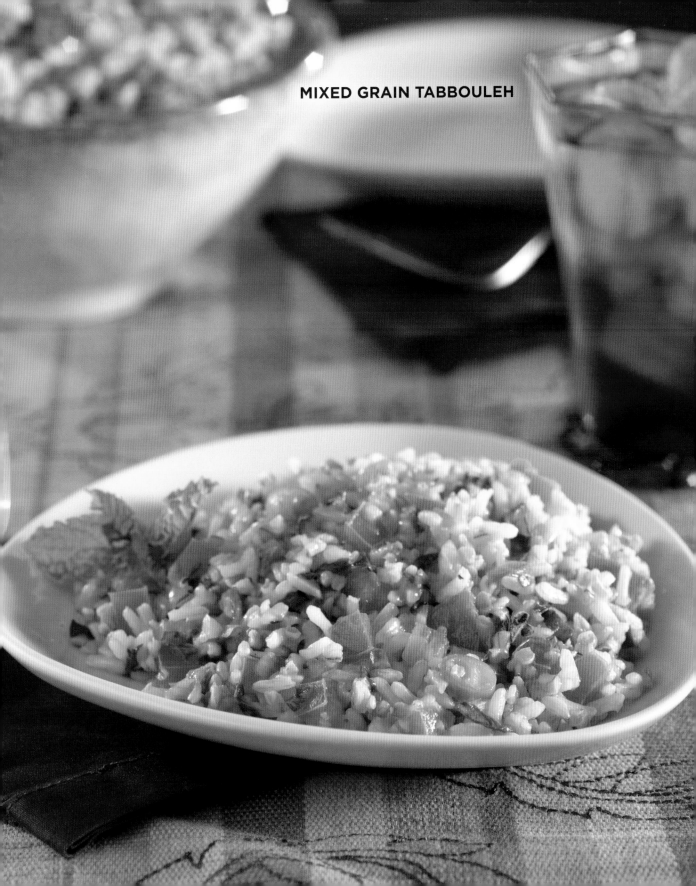

Quinoa Burrito Bowls

1 cup uncooked quinoa

2 cups water

¾ teaspoon salt, divided

2 tablespoons lime juice, divided

2 teaspoons vegetable oil

1 small onion, diced

1 red bell pepper, diced

1 clove garlic, minced

½ cup canned black beans, rinsed and drained

½ cup thawed frozen corn

¼ cup sour cream

Shredded lettuce

Lime wedges (optional)

1. Place quinoa in fine-mesh strainer; rinse well under cold running water. Combine quinoa, 2 cups water and ½ teaspoon salt in medium saucepan; bring to a boil over high heat. Reduce heat to low; cover and simmer 15 to 18 minutes or until quinoa is tender and water is absorbed. Stir in 1 tablespoon lime juice. Cover and keep warm.

2. Meanwhile, heat oil in large skillet over medium heat. Add onion and bell pepper; cook and stir 5 minutes or until softened. Add garlic; cook and stir 1 minute. Add beans, corn and remaining ¼ teaspoon salt; cook 3 to 5 minutes or until heated through, stirring occasionally.

3. Combine sour cream and remaining 1 tablespoon lime juice in small bowl; mix well.

4. Divide quinoa among four serving bowls; top with bean mixture, lettuce and sour cream mixture. Garnish with lime wedges.

Makes 4 servings

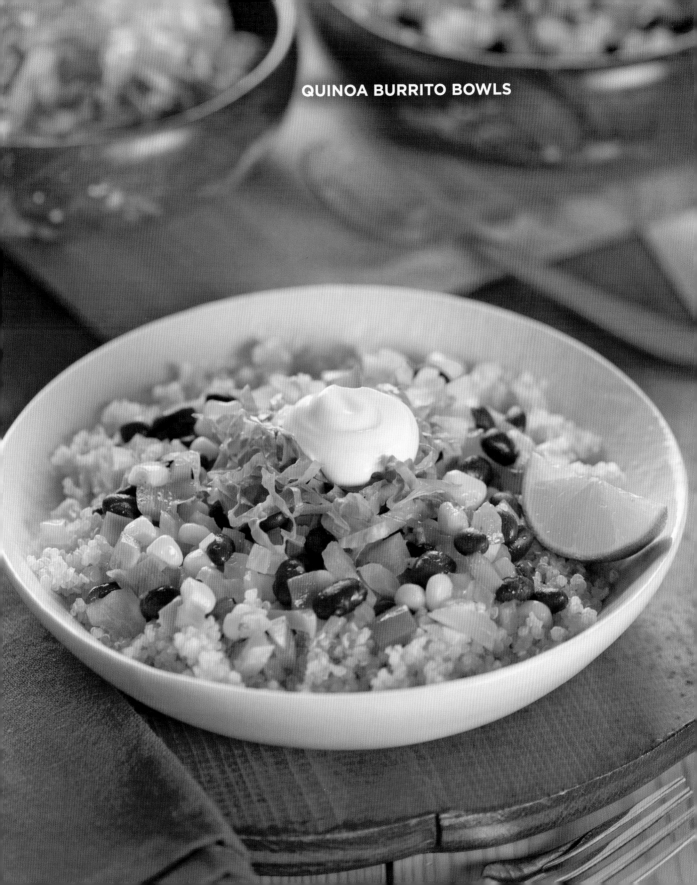

QUINOA BURRITO BOWLS

Roasted Beet Risotto

2 medium beets, trimmed

1 container (32 ounces) reduced-sodium vegetable broth, divided

1 tablespoon olive oil

1 cup uncooked Arborio rice

1 medium leek, white and light green parts only, finely chopped

½ cup crumbled goat cheese, plus additional for garnish

1 teaspoon Italian seasoning

¼ teaspoon salt

Juice of 1 lemon

Lemon wedges (optional)

1. Preheat oven to 400°F. Wrap each beet tightly with foil; place on baking sheet. Roast 45 minutes to 1 hour or until knife inserted into centers goes in easily. Unwrap beets; let stand 15 minutes or until cool enough to handle. Peel and cut beets into bite-size pieces. Set aside.

2. Bring broth to a simmer in medium saucepan; keep warm over low heat.

3. Heat oil in separate medium saucepan over medium-high heat. Add rice; cook and stir 1 to 2 minutes. Add leek; cook and stir 1 to 2 minutes. Add broth, ½ cup at a time, stirring constantly until broth is absorbed before adding next ½ cup. Continue adding broth and stirring until rice is tender and mixture is creamy, about 20 to 25 minutes. Remove from heat.

4. Add ½ cup cheese, Italian seasoning and salt; mix well. Gently stir in beets. Sprinkle with lemon juice and additional cheese, if desired. Garnish with lemon wedges. Serve immediately.

Makes 4 servings

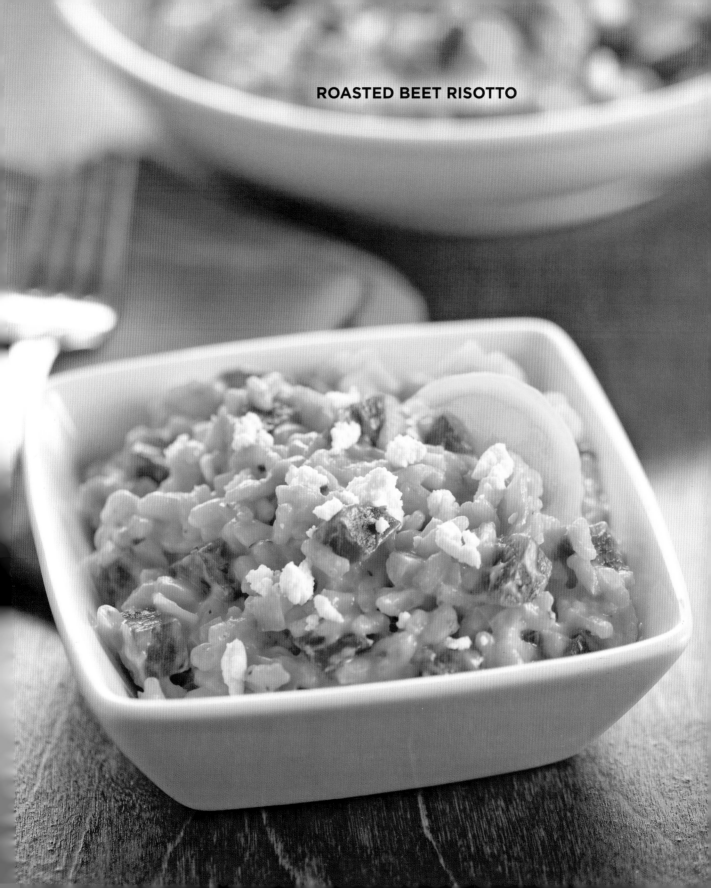

ROASTED BEET RISOTTO

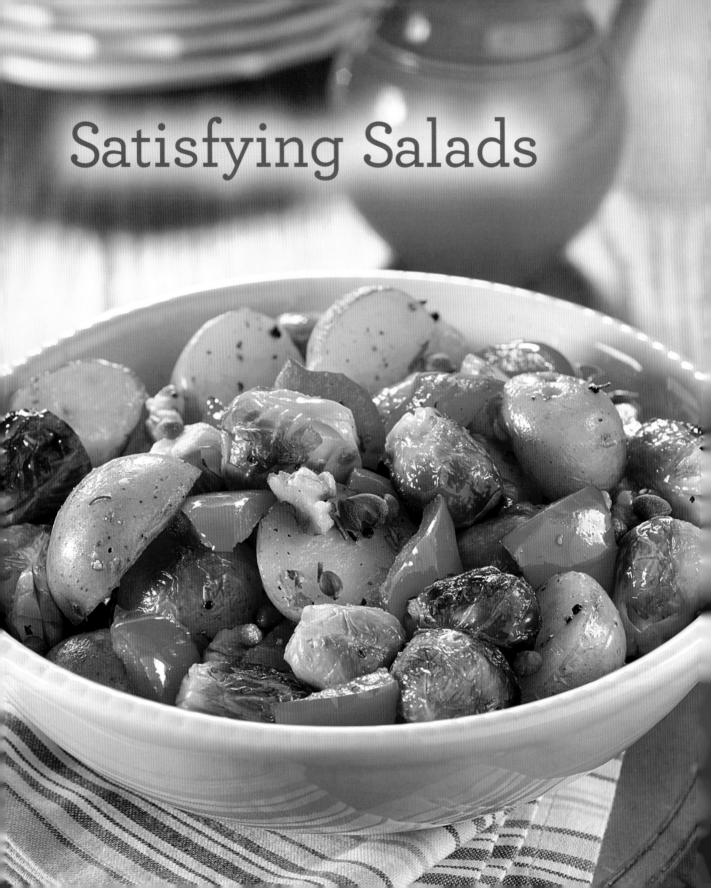

Satisfying Salads

Roasted Vegetable Salad with Capers and Walnuts

- 1 pound small brussels sprouts, trimmed
- 1 pound unpeeled small Yukon Gold potatoes, cut into halves
- ½ teaspoon salt
- ¼ teaspoon black pepper
- ¼ teaspoon dried rosemary
- 5 tablespoons olive oil, divided
- 1 red bell pepper, cut into bite-size pieces
- ¼ cup walnuts, coarsely chopped
- 2 tablespoons capers, drained
- 1½ tablespoons white wine vinegar

1. Preheat oven to 400°F.

2. Slash bottoms of brussels sprouts; place on baking sheet. Add potatoes; sprinkle with salt, black pepper and rosemary. Drizzle with 3 tablespoons oil; toss to coat. Spread vegetables in single layer.

3. Roast 20 minutes. Stir in bell pepper; roast 15 minutes or until tender. Transfer to large bowl; stir in walnuts and capers.

4. Whisk remaining 2 tablespoons oil and vinegar in small bowl until blended. Pour over vegetable mixture; toss to coat. Serve at room temperature.

Makes 6 to 8 servings

Greek Rice Salad

    1 cup water
    ¾ cup uncooked instant brown rice
    1 cup packed baby spinach
    ⅔ cup quartered cherry tomatoes
    1 tablespoon lemon juice
    1 tablespoon extra virgin olive oil
 1½ teaspoons Greek seasoning
    ½ teaspoon salt
    ⅛ teaspoon black pepper
    ¼ cup pine nuts

1. Bring water to a boil in small saucepan over high heat. Add rice; return to a boil. Reduce heat to low; cover and simmer 5 minutes. Remove from heat; let stand 5 minutes. Rinse rice under cold water until cool; drain.

2. Combine spinach, tomatoes and rice in medium bowl; mix well. Whisk lemon juice, oil, Greek seasoning, salt and pepper in small bowl until well blended.

3. Pour dressing over spinach mixture; toss to coat. Serve immediately or refrigerate until ready to serve. Sprinkle with pine nuts.

Makes 4 servings

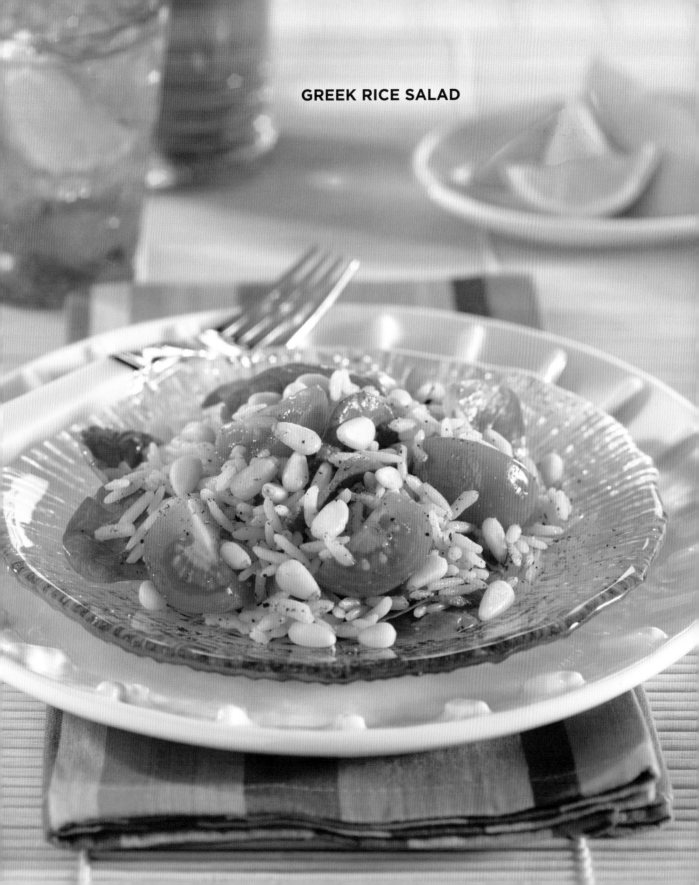

GREEK RICE SALAD

Farmers' Market Potato Salad

Pickled Red Onions (recipe follows)

2 cups cubed unpeeled potatoes (purple, baby red, Yukon Gold and/or a combination)

1 cup green beans, cut into 1-inch pieces

2 tablespoons plain Greek yogurt

2 tablespoons white wine vinegar

2 tablespoons olive oil

1 tablespoon spicy mustard

1 teaspoon salt

1. Prepare Pickled Red Onions.

2. Bring large saucepan of water to a boil over medium-high heat. Add potatoes; cook 5 to 8 minutes or until fork-tender.* Add green beans during last 4 minutes of cooking time. Drain potatoes and beans.

3. Whisk yogurt, vinegar, oil, mustard and salt in large bowl until well blended.

4. Add potatoes, beans and pickled onions to dressing; gently toss to coat. Cover and refrigerate at least 1 hour before serving.

*Some potatoes may take longer to cook than others. Remove individual potatoes to large bowl with slotted spoon when fork-tender.

Makes 6 servings

Pickled Red Onions: Combine ½ cup thinly sliced red onion, ¼ cup white wine vinegar, 2 tablespoons water, 1 teaspoon sugar and ½ teaspoon salt in large glass jar. Seal jar; shake well. Refrigerate at least 1 hour or up to 1 week.

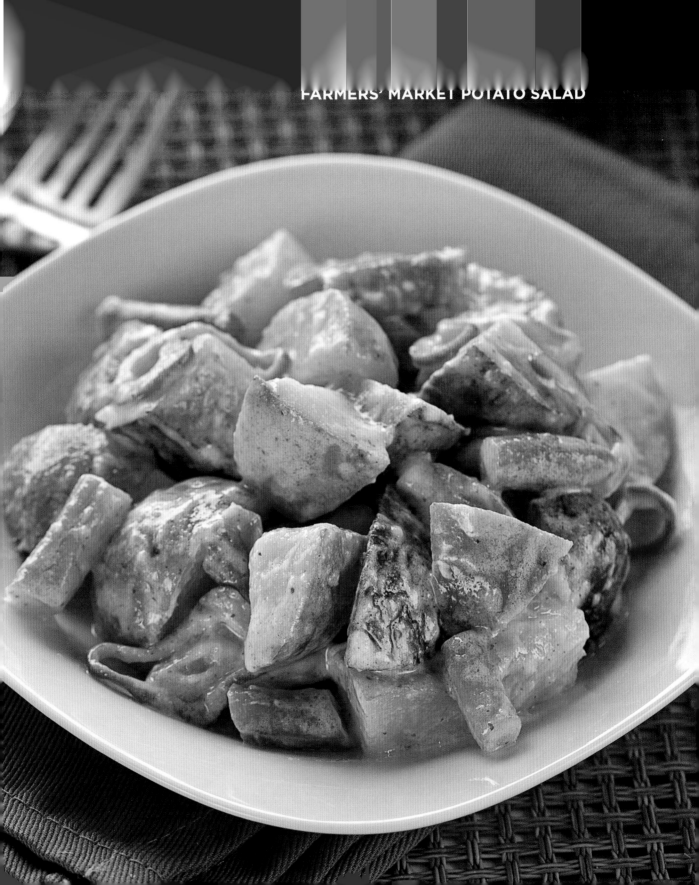

Spinach Salad with Pomegranate Vinaigrette

  1 **package (5 ounces) baby spinach**
  ½ **cup pomegranate seeds (arils)**
  ¼ **cup crumbled goat cheese**
  2 **tablespoons chopped walnuts, toasted***
  ¼ **cup pomegranate juice**
  2 **tablespoons olive oil**
  1 **tablespoon red wine vinegar**
  1 **tablespoon honey**
  ¼ **teaspoon salt**
  ¼ **teaspoon black pepper**

* To toast walnuts, cook in heavy skillet over medium heat 1 to 2 minutes, stirring frequently, until nuts are fragrant. Immediately remove from skillet; cool before using.

1. Combine spinach, pomegranate seeds, goat cheese and walnuts in large bowl.
2. Whisk pomegranate juice, oil, vinegar, honey, salt and pepper in small bowl until well blended. Pour over salad; toss gently to coat. Serve immediately.

Makes 4 servings

Tip: For easier removal of pomegranate seeds, cut a pomegranate into pieces and immerse in a bowl of cold water. The membrane that holds the seeds in place will float to the top; discard it and collect the seeds. For convenience, you can find containers of ready-to-use pomegranate seeds in the refrigerated produce section of some supermarkets.

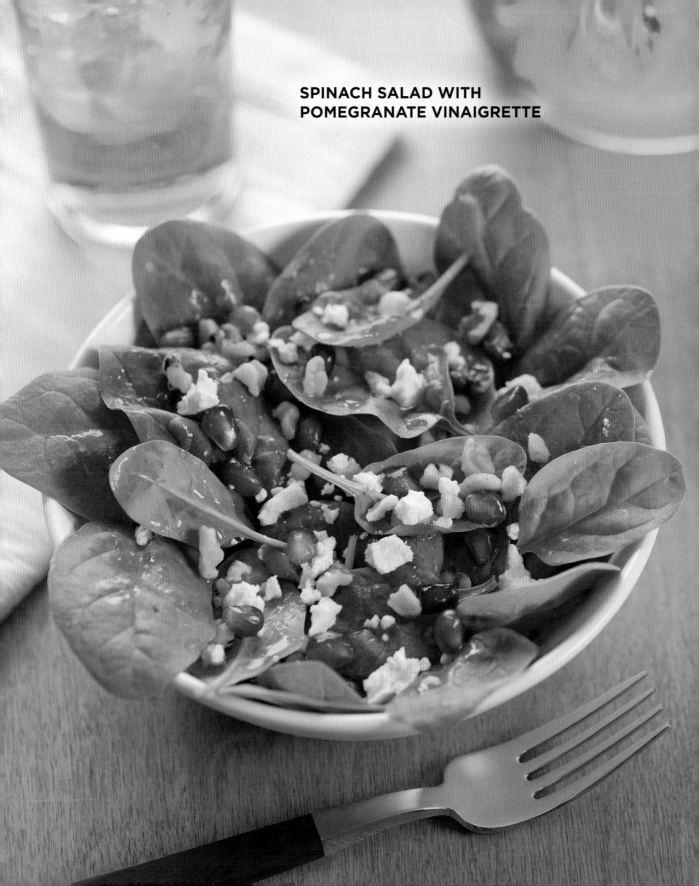

SPINACH SALAD WITH
POMEGRANATE VINAIGRETTE

Quinoa and Mango Salad

1 cup uncooked quinoa

2 cups water

2 cups cubed peeled mangoes (about 2 large)

½ cup sliced green onions

½ cup dried cranberries

2 tablespoons chopped fresh parsley

¼ cup extra virgin olive oil

1½ tablespoons white wine vinegar

1 teaspoon Dijon mustard

½ teaspoon salt

⅛ teaspoon black pepper

1. Place quinoa in fine-mesh strainer; rinse well under cold running water. Combine quinoa and 2 cups water in medium saucepan; bring to a boil over high heat. Reduce heat to low; cover and simmer 12 to 15 minutes until quinoa is tender and water is absorbed. Stir quinoa; let stand, covered, 15 minutes. Transfer to large bowl; cover and refrigerate at least 1 hour.

2. Add mangoes, green onions, cranberries and parsley to quinoa; mix well.

3. Whisk oil, vinegar, mustard, salt and pepper in small bowl until blended. Pour over quinoa mixture; mix well.

Makes 6 to 8 servings

Tip: This salad can be made several hours ahead and refrigerated. Let stand at room temperature at least 30 minutes before serving.

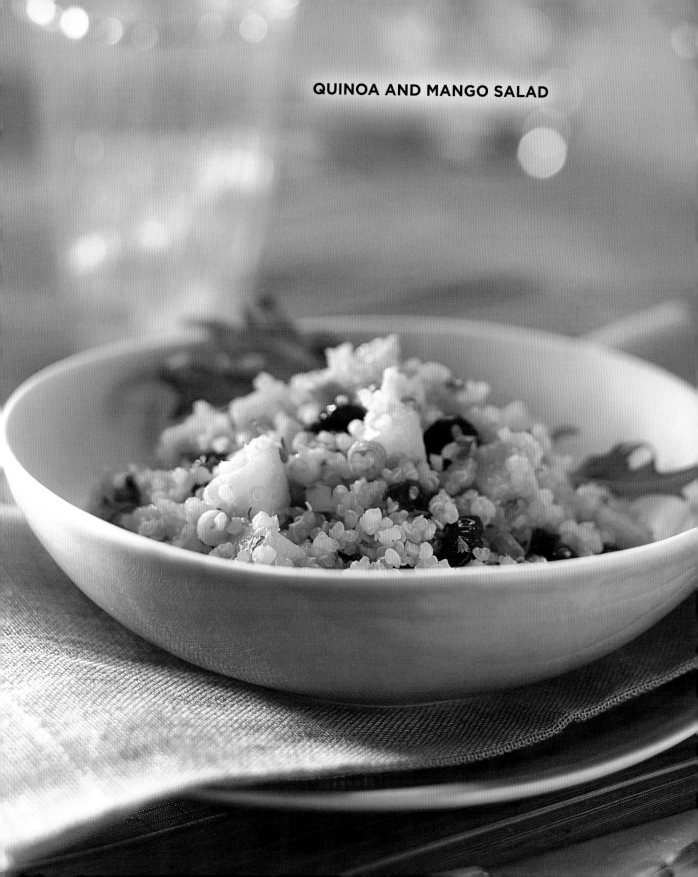

Orzo Salad with Zucchini and Feta

½ cup uncooked orzo pasta

1½ tablespoons extra virgin olive oil, divided

1 cup coarsely chopped zucchini

½ cup finely chopped fresh Italian parsley

⅓ cup thinly sliced radishes

⅓ cup crumbled feta cheese

2 tablespoons thinly sliced green onion

1 tablespoon lemon juice

¼ teaspoon salt

⅛ teaspoon black pepper

1. Cook orzo according to package directions; drain and rinse under cold water. Drain well and transfer to large bowl.

2. Meanwhile heat ½ tablespoon oil in medium skillet over medium-high heat. Add zucchini; cook and stir 3 minutes or until crisp-tender. Add to orzo with parsley, radishes, cheese and green onion.

3. Whisk remaining 1 tablespoon oil, lemon juice, salt and pepper in small bowl until well blended. Pour over orzo mixture; toss gently to coat.

Makes 4 servings

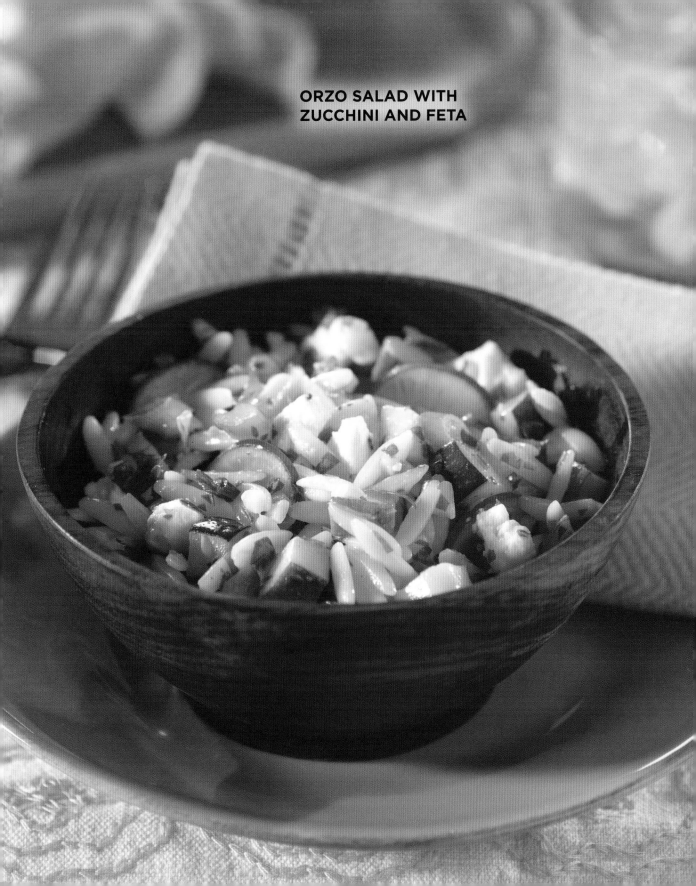

ORZO SALAD WITH ZUCCHINI AND FETA

Classic Irish Salad

Dressing

3 tablespoons mayonnaise

1 tablespoon Dijon mustard

1 tablespoon canola oil

1 tablespoon cider vinegar

2 teaspoons sugar

¼ teaspoon salt

⅛ teaspoon black pepper

Salad

6 cups torn romaine lettuce

2 cups baby arugula

1 large cucumber, halved lengthwise and sliced

4 radishes, thinly sliced

3 tablespoons chopped fresh chives

2 hard-cooked eggs, cut into wedges

2 bottled pickled beets, quartered

1. For dressing, whisk mayonnaise, mustard, oil, vinegar, sugar, salt and pepper in small bowl until well blended.

2. For salad, toss romaine, arugula, cucumber, radishes and chives in large bowl. Divide among four plates; top with egg wedges and beet quarters. Serve dressing separately or drizzle over salads just before serving.

Makes 4 servings

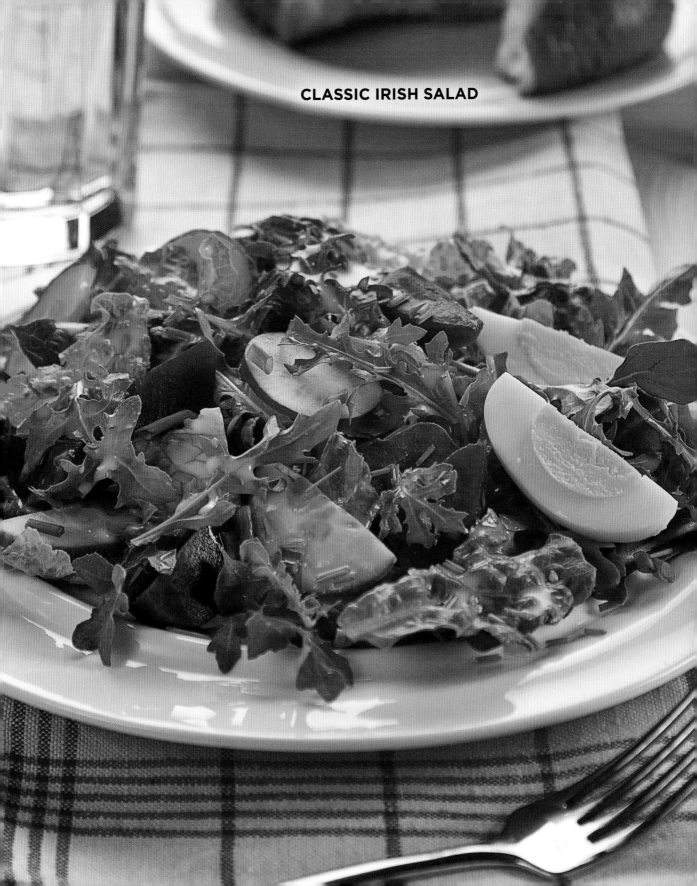

CLASSIC IRISH SALAD

Southwestern Chile Bean Salad

  2 cups canned pinto beans, rinsed and drained

  2 medium tomatoes, diced

  ½ cup chopped green onions

  1 large stalk celery, thinly sliced

  1 jalapeño pepper,* seeded and minced

  2 tablespoons tomato juice

  4 teaspoons red wine vinegar

  1 tablespoon canola oil

  ½ teaspoon paprika

  ¼ teaspoon ground cumin

  ¼ teaspoon salt

  ¼ teaspoon black pepper

  ½ cup (2 ounces) shredded sharp Cheddar cheese

Jalapeño peppers can sting and irritate the skin, so wear rubber gloves when handling peppers and do not touch your eyes.

1. Combine beans, tomatoes, green onions, celery and jalapeño in large bowl; mix gently.

2. Whisk tomato juice, vinegar, oil, paprika, cumin, salt and black pepper in small bowl until well blended. Pour over salad; toss gently to coat. Sprinkle with cheese.

Makes 4 servings

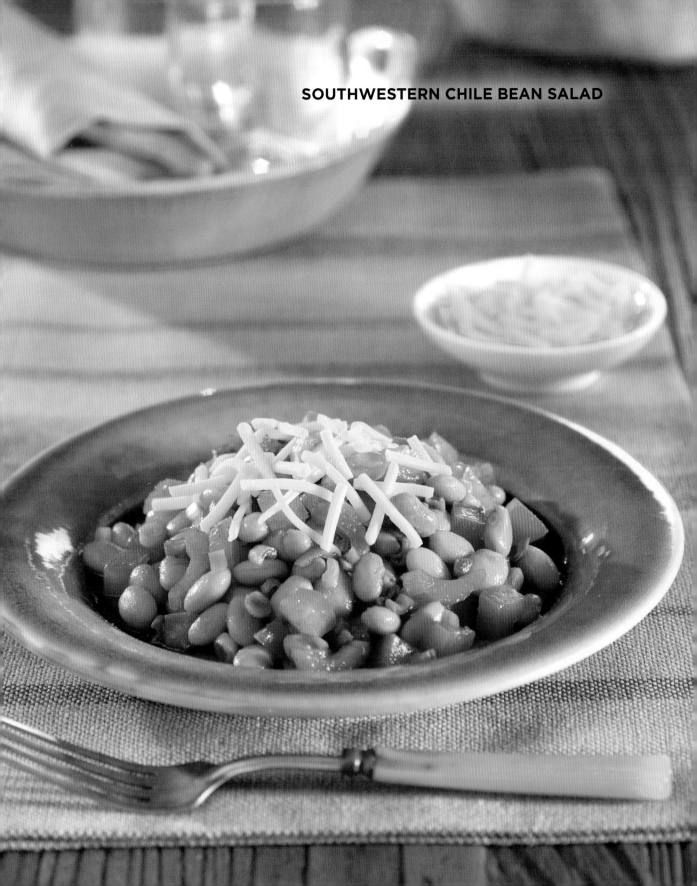

SOUTHWESTERN CHILE BEAN SALAD

Zesty Zucchini Chickpea Salad

3 medium zucchini

½ teaspoon salt

5 tablespoons white vinegar

1 clove garlic, minced

¼ teaspoon dried thyme

½ cup olive oil

1 cup canned chickpeas, rinsed and drained

½ cup sliced pitted black olives

3 green onions, minced

1 canned chipotle pepper in adobo sauce, drained, seeded and minced

1 ripe avocado

⅓ cup crumbled feta cheese *or* 3 tablespoons grated Romano cheese

Boston lettuce leaves

Sliced tomato and fresh cilantro sprigs (optional)

1. Cut zucchini lengthwise into halves; cut halves crosswise into ¼-inch-thick slices. Place slices in medium bowl; sprinkle with salt and mix well. Spread zucchini on several layers of paper towels. Let stand at room temperature 30 minutes to drain.

2. Combine vinegar, garlic and thyme in large bowl. Gradually whisk in oil until well blended. Pat zucchini dry; add to dressing. Add chickpeas, olives and green onions; toss gently to coat. Cover and refrigerate at least 30 minutes or up to 4 hours, stirring occasionally.

3. Stir in chipotle pepper just before serving. Cut avocado into ½-inch cubes. Add avocado and cheese to salad; toss gently. Serve salad over lettuce; garnish with tomato and cilantro.

Makes 4 to 6 servings

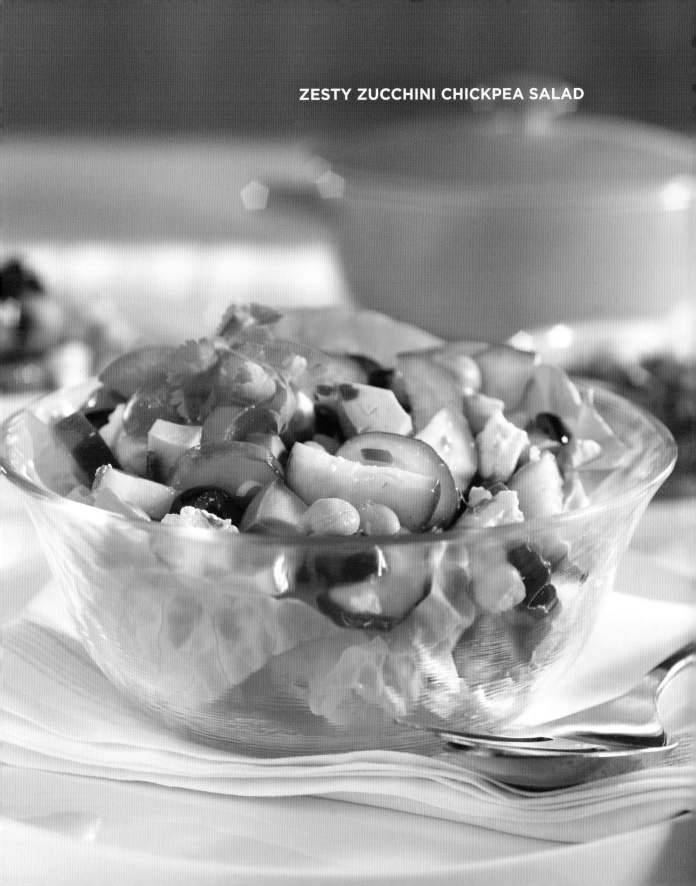

Toasted Peanut Couscous Salad

½ cup water

¼ cup uncooked couscous

1 ounce dry-roasted peanuts

½ cup finely chopped red onion

½ cup finely chopped green bell pepper

1 tablespoon reduced-sodium soy sauce

2 teaspoons cider vinegar

1½ teaspoons sesame oil

½ teaspoon grated fresh ginger

1 teaspoon sugar

¼ teaspoon salt

⅛ teaspoon red pepper flakes

1. Bring water to boil in small saucepan over high heat. Remove from heat; stir in couscous. Let stand, covered, 5 minutes or until water is absorbed.

2. Heat small skillet over medium-high heat. Add peanuts; cook 2 to 3 minutes or until nuts begin to turn golden, stirring frequently.

3. Combine onion, bell pepper, soy sauce, vinegar, oil, ginger, sugar, salt and red pepper flakes in medium bowl; mix well. Add couscous and toasted nuts; toss gently.

Makes 4 servings

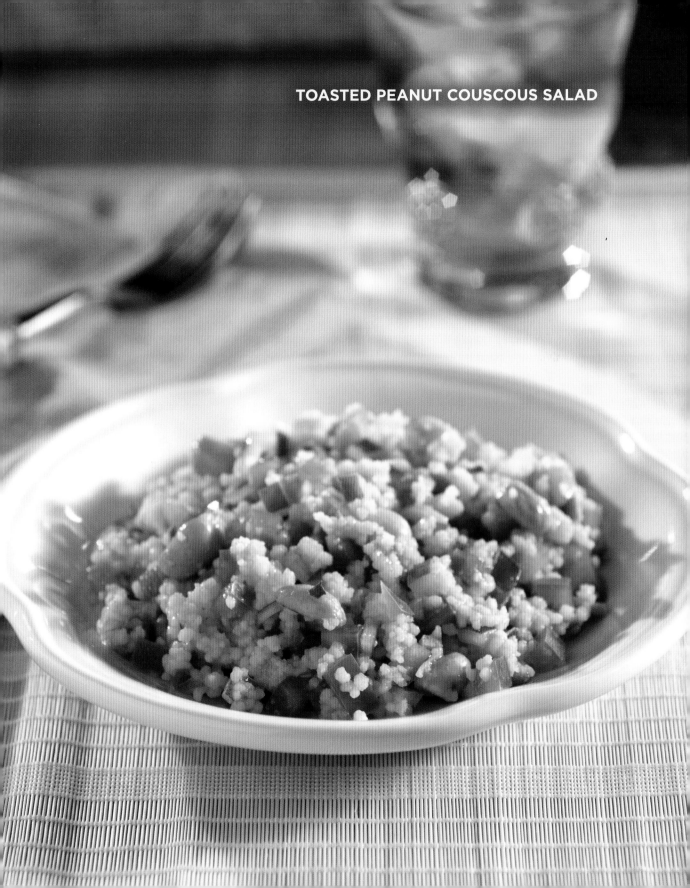

Layered Mexican Salad

   1 package (10 ounces) shredded lettuce
   ½ cup chopped green onions
   ½ cup sour cream
   ⅓ cup medium picante sauce
   1 medium lime, halved
   1 teaspoon sugar
   ½ teaspoon ground cumin
   ¼ teaspoon salt
   1 medium avocado, chopped
   ¾ cup (3 ounces) shredded sharp Cheddar cheese
   2 ounces tortilla chips, coarsely crumbled

1. Place lettuce in 13×9-inch baking dish. Sprinkle with green onions.

2. Whisk sour cream, picante sauce, juice from half of lime, sugar, cumin and salt in small bowl until well blended.

3. Spoon sour cream mixture over lettuce and green onions; top with avocado. Squeeze remaining lime half over avocado layer. Sprinkle with cheese.

4. Cover with plastic wrap; refrigerate until ready to serve. (Salad may be prepared up to 8 hours in advance, if desired.) Sprinkle with crumbled tortilla chips just before serving.

Makes 8 servings

Variation: Add chopped fresh tomatoes to the avocado layer. Sprinkle with chopped fresh cilantro.

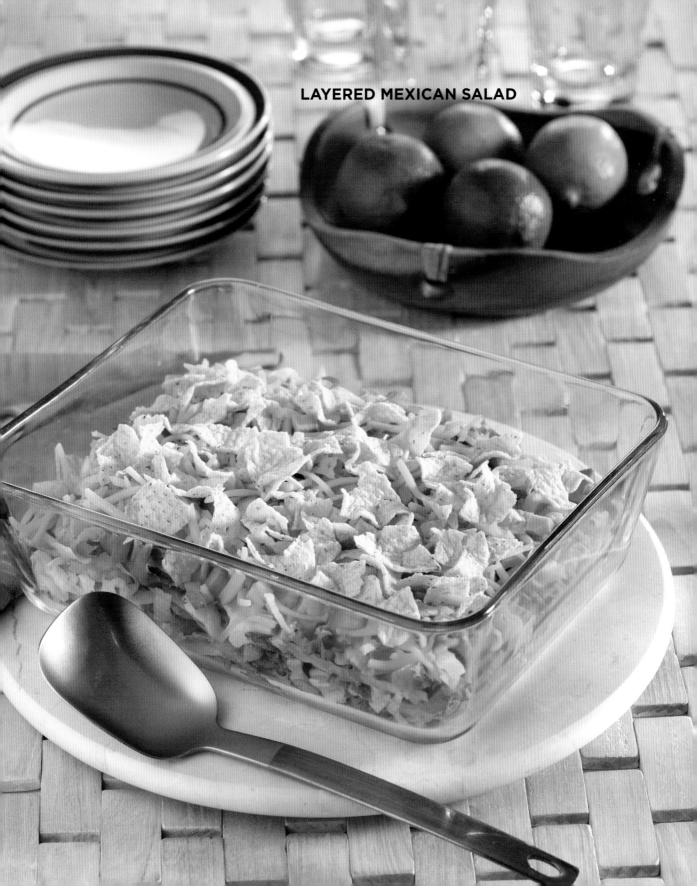

LAYERED MEXICAN SALAD

Asian Tofu Salad

½ package (16 ounces) extra firm tofu, drained

4 tablespoons rice vinegar

3 tablespoons reduced-sodium soy sauce

1½ tablespoons sugar

1 tablespoon dark sesame oil or canola oil

1 teaspoon grated fresh ginger

1 teaspoon Chinese chili-garlic sauce

1 cup snow peas, trimmed

8 cups mixed salad greens

2 medium carrots, julienned

1 medium cucumber, thinly sliced

¼ cup dry roasted peanuts, coarsely chopped (optional)

1. Cut tofu into ½-inch cubes, place in single layer on kitchen towel.

2. Whisk vinegar, soy sauce, sugar, oil, ginger and chili-garlic sauce in small bowl until well blended.

3. Combine tofu, 2 tablespoons soy sauce mixture and snow peas in medium nonstick skillet over medium-high heat; cook and stir 5 to 7 minutes. Cool slightly.

4. Combine mixed greens, carrots and cucumber in large bowl. Drizzle with remaining soy sauce mixture; toss to coat.

5. Top with warm tofu mixture and peanuts, if desired. Serve immediately.

Makes 4 to 6 servings

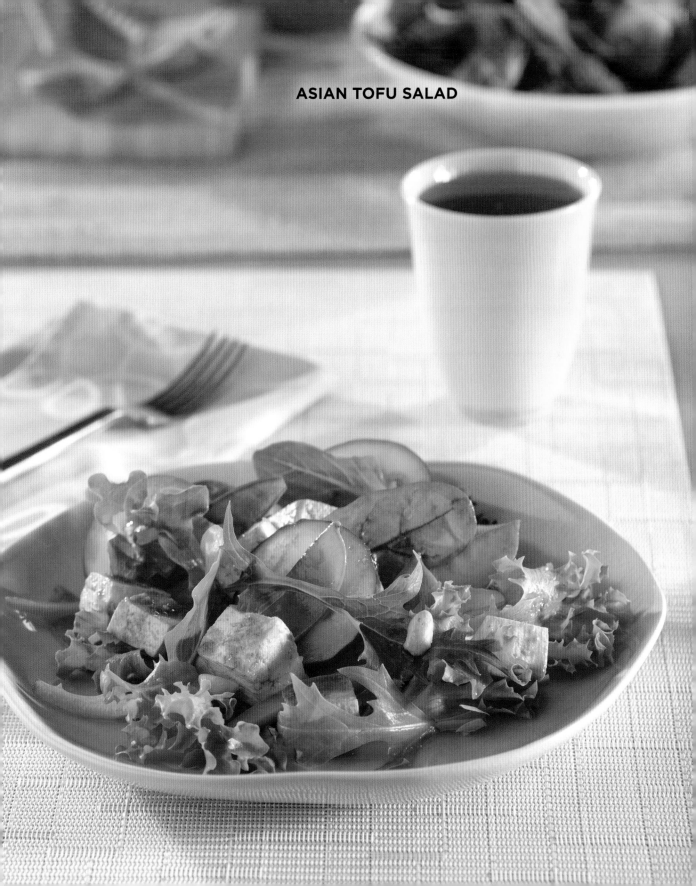

ASIAN TOFU SALAD

Orange Twisted Quinoa Waldorf Salad

½ cup uncooked quinoa

1 cup water

½ teaspoon salt, divided

½ cup quartered seedless grapes (green, red or a combination)

1 small apple, chopped

1 stalk celery, chopped

¼ cup chopped walnuts, toasted*

¼ cup plain Greek yogurt

2 tablespoons orange juice

1½ teaspoons honey

Dash black pepper

1 cup canned mandarin oranges, drained

Fresh mint leaves (optional)

To toast walnuts, cook in small heavy skillet over medium heat 2 to 3 minutes or until fragrant, stirring frequently. Immediately remove from skillet; cool completely before using.

1. Place quinoa in fine-mesh strainer; rinse well under cold running water. Combine quinoa, 1 cup water and ¼ teaspoon salt in small saucepan; bring to a boil over high heat. Reduce heat to low; cover and simmer 12 to 15 minutes or until quinoa is tender and water is absorbed.

2. Transfer quinoa to large bowl. Stir in grapes, apple, celery and walnuts.

3. Whisk yogurt, orange juice, honey, remaining ¼ teaspoon salt and pepper in small bowl until well blended Add to quinoa mixture; mix well. Add orange sections; toss gently. Garnish with mint.

Makes 4 servings

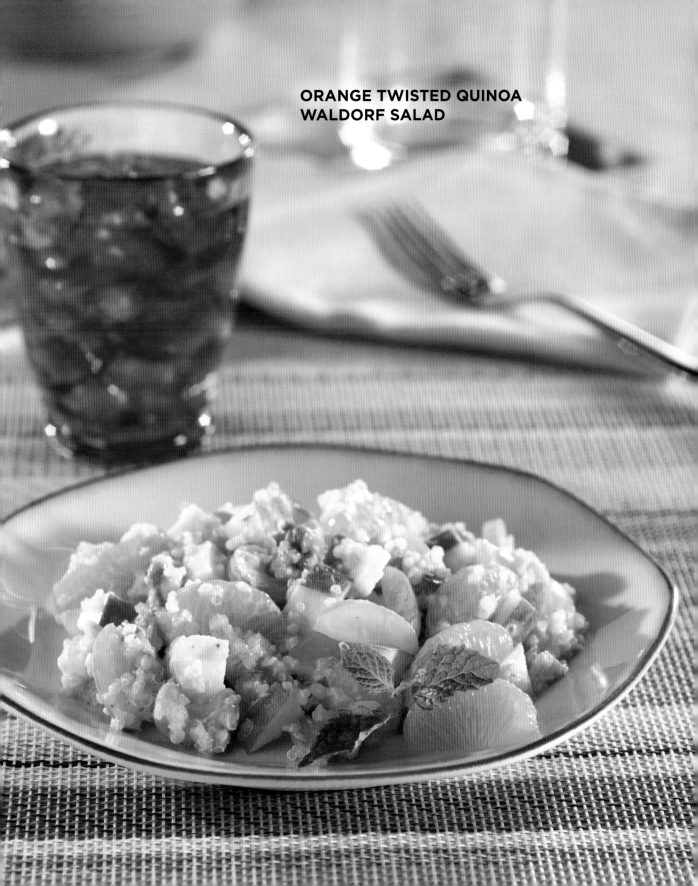

ORANGE TWISTED QUINOA WALDORF SALAD

Spiced Rice and Carrot Salad

⅔ cup cold cooked brown rice

2 medium carrots, shredded

1 green onion, chopped

2 teaspoons canola oil

1 teaspoon white wine vinegar

1 teaspoon Chinese chili-garlic sauce

¼ teaspoon salt

⅛ teaspoon black pepper

1. Combine rice, carrots and green onion in medium bowl. Whisk oil, vinegar, chili-garlic sauce, salt and pepper in small bowl until well blended.

2. Add dressing to rice mixture; mix well.

Makes 2 servings

Black Bean Mexicali Salad

1 can (about 15 ounces) black beans, rinsed and drained

1 cup fresh or thawed frozen corn

6 ounces roasted red bell peppers, cut into thin strips

½ cup chopped red or yellow onion

⅓ cup mild chipotle or regular salsa

2 tablespoons cider vinegar

2 ounces mozzarella cheese, cut into ¼-inch cubes

Chopped fresh cilantro (optional)

1. Combine beans, corn, roasted peppers, onion, salsa and vinegar in medium bowl; mix well. Let stand 15 minutes.

2. Just before serving, gently fold in cheese. Garnish with cilantro.

Makes 6 servings

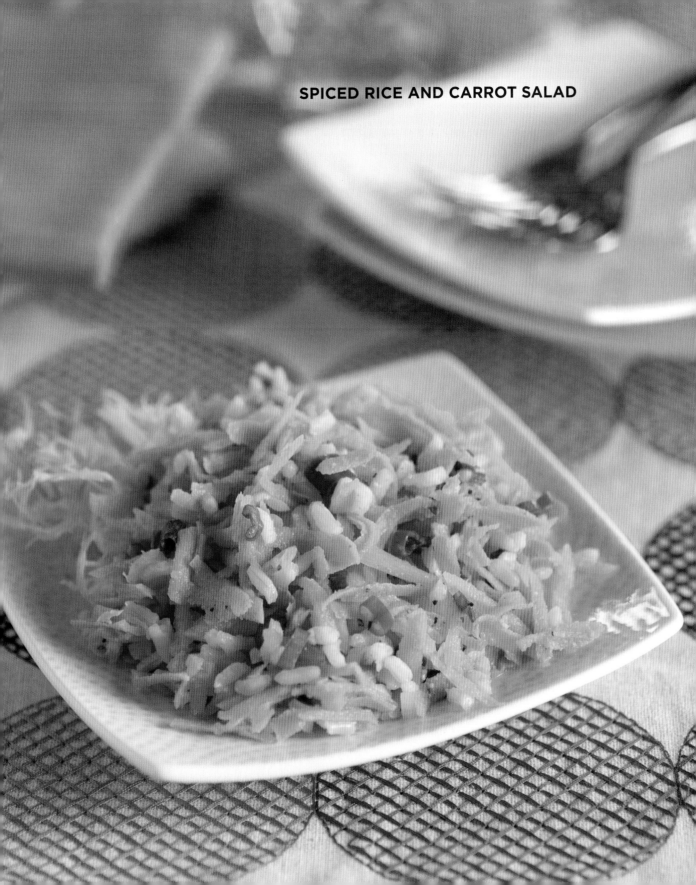

SPICED RICE AND CARROT SALAD

Cold Peanut Noodle and Edamame Salad

½ (8-ounce) package brown rice pad thai noodles*

3 tablespoons reduced-sodium soy sauce

2 tablespoons toasted sesame oil

2 tablespoons unseasoned rice vinegar

1 tablespoon sugar

1 tablespoon finely grated fresh ginger

1 tablespoon creamy peanut butter

1 tablespoon sriracha or hot chili sauce

2 teaspoons minced garlic

½ cup thawed frozen shelled edamame

¼ cup shredded carrots

¼ cup sliced green onions

   Chopped peanuts

*Brown rice pad thai noodles can be found in the Asian section of the supermarket. Or substitute 4 ounces whole wheat spaghetti for the rice noodles.

1. Prepare noodles according to package directions for pasta. Rinse under cold water; drain. Cut noodles into 3-inch lengths; place in large bowl.

2. Whisk soy sauce, oil, vinegar, sugar, ginger, peanut butter, sriracha and garlic in small bowl until well blended.

3. Add dressing to noodles; toss gently to coat. Stir in edamame and carrots. Cover and refrigerate at least 30 minutes before serving. Top with green onions and peanuts.

Makes 4 servings

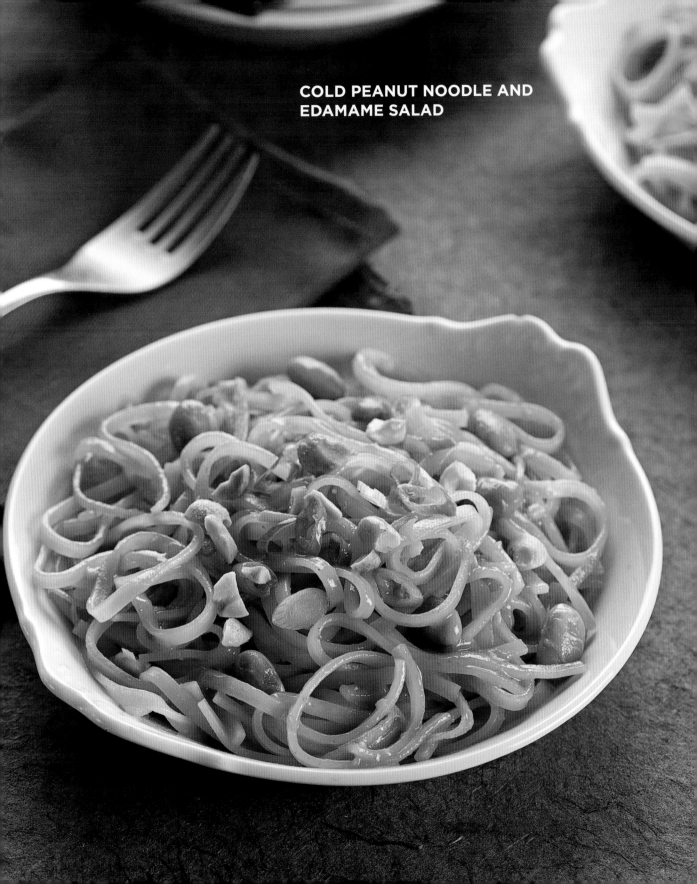

COLD PEANUT NOODLE AND
EDAMAME SALAD

Veggie Salad with White Beans and Feta

   1 can (about 15 ounces) navy beans, rinsed and drained

   1 can (14 ounces) quartered artichoke hearts, drained

   1 medium green bell pepper, chopped

   1 yellow bell pepper, chopped

   1 cup grape tomatoes, halved

   ¼ cup chopped fresh basil

   ¼ cup extra virgin olive oil

   3 to 4 tablespoons red wine vinegar

   1 clove garlic, minced

   1 teaspoon Dijon mustard

   ½ teaspoon black pepper

   ¼ teaspoon salt

   1 package (4 ounces) crumbled feta cheese with sun-dried tomatoes
      and basil

   1 package (about 5 ounces) spring greens mix

1. Combine beans, artichokes, bell peppers, tomatoes, basil, oil, vinegar, garlic, mustard, pepper and salt in large bowl; toss gently. Fold in cheese. Let stand 10 minutes.

2. Place greens on serving plates; top with vegetable mixture.

Makes 4 servings

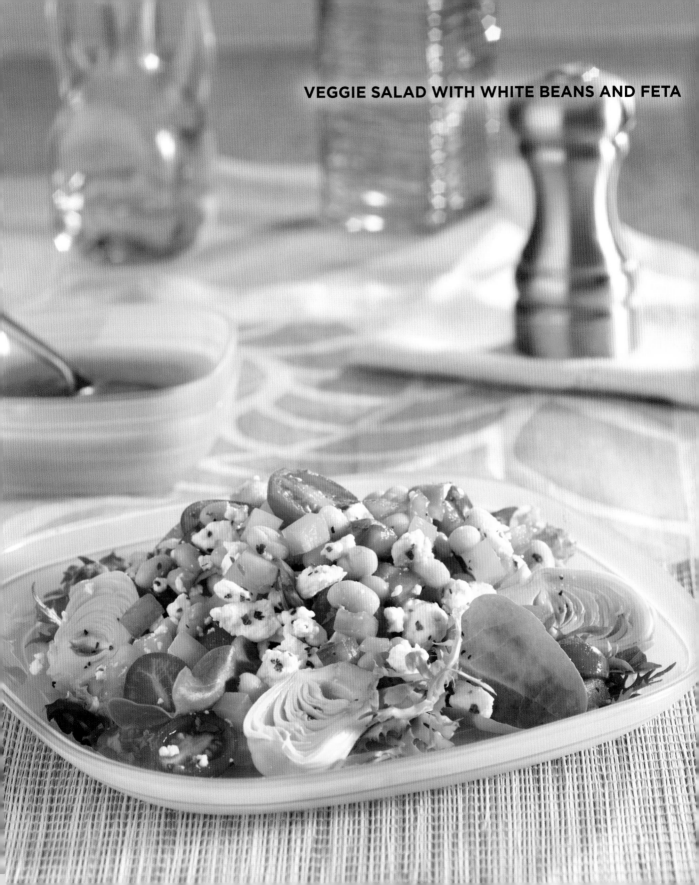

VEGGIE SALAD WITH WHITE BEANS AND FETA

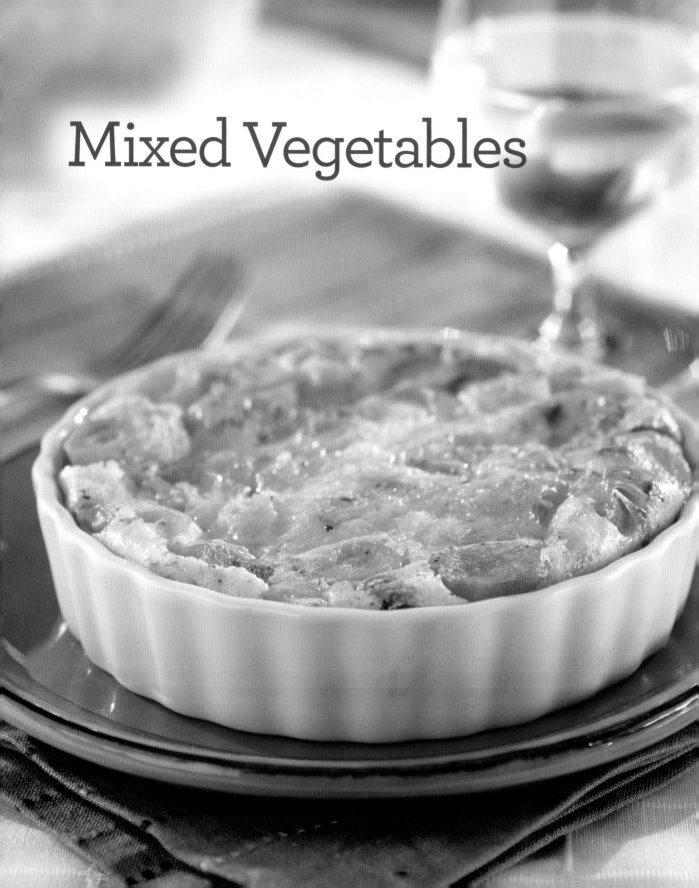

Mixed Vegetables

French Carrot Quiche

- 1 tablespoon butter, plus additional for baking dishes
- 1 pound carrots, peeled and sliced
- ¼ cup chopped green onions
- ½ teaspoon herbes de Provence
- 1 cup milk
- ¼ cup whipping cream
- ½ cup all-purpose flour
- 2 eggs, lightly beaten
- ½ teaspoon minced fresh thyme
- ¼ teaspoon ground nutmeg
- ½ cup (2 ounces) shredded Gruyère or Swiss cheese

1. Preheat oven to 350°F. Butter four shallow 1-cup baking dishes or one 9-inch quiche dish or shallow casserole.

2. Melt 1 tablespoon butter in large skillet over medium heat. Add carrots, green onions and herbes de Provence; cook and stir 3 to 4 minutes or until carrots are tender.

3. Meanwhile, combine milk and cream in medium bowl; gradually whisk in flour until well blended. Beat in eggs, thyme and nutmeg.

4. Spread carrot mixture in prepared baking dishes. Pour in milk mixture; sprinkle with cheese.

5. Bake 20 to 25 minutes for individual quiches or 30 to 40 minutes for 9-inch quiche or until firm. Serve warm or at room temperature.

Makes 4 servings

Butternut Gnocchi with Herb Butter

1 butternut squash (about 2½ pounds), peeled, seeded and cut into 1-inch pieces

1 cup rice flour, plus additional for work surface

3½ teaspoons salt, divided

1 teaspoon xanthan gum

¼ teaspoon black pepper

4 quarts water

¼ cup (½ stick) butter

2 teaspoons minced garlic

1 teaspoon dried parsley flakes

1 teaspoon rubbed sage

½ teaspoon dried thyme

Juice of 1 lemon

¼ cup shredded Parmesan cheese

1. Place squash in large microwavable bowl; cover with vented plastic wrap. Microwave on HIGH 6 to 7 minutes or until very tender. Let stand 10 minutes to cool slightly. Drain.

2. Mash squash or press through ricer into medium bowl. Add 1 cup rice flour, 2 teaspoons salt, xanthan gum and pepper; mix well.

3. Heavily dust cutting board or work surface with rice flour. Working in batches, scoop portions of dough onto board and roll into ½-inch-thick rope using rice-floured hands. Cut each rope into ¾-inch pieces.

4. Bring water and 1 teaspoon salt to a boil in large saucepan over high heat. Drop 8 to 12 gnocchi into boiling water; cook about 2½ minutes or until gnocchi float to surface. Remove gnocchi with slotted spoon; drain on paper towel-lined plate. Return water to a boil; repeat with remaining gnocchi.

5. Combine butter, garlic, parsley flakes, sage, thyme and remaining ½ teaspoon salt in large nonstick skillet; heat over medium heat until butter is melted and just begins to brown. Add lemon juice; cook 30 seconds. Add gnocchi; gently toss to coat. Cook 2 minutes or until lightly browned and heated through. Sprinkle with cheese. Serve immediately.

Makes 4 servings

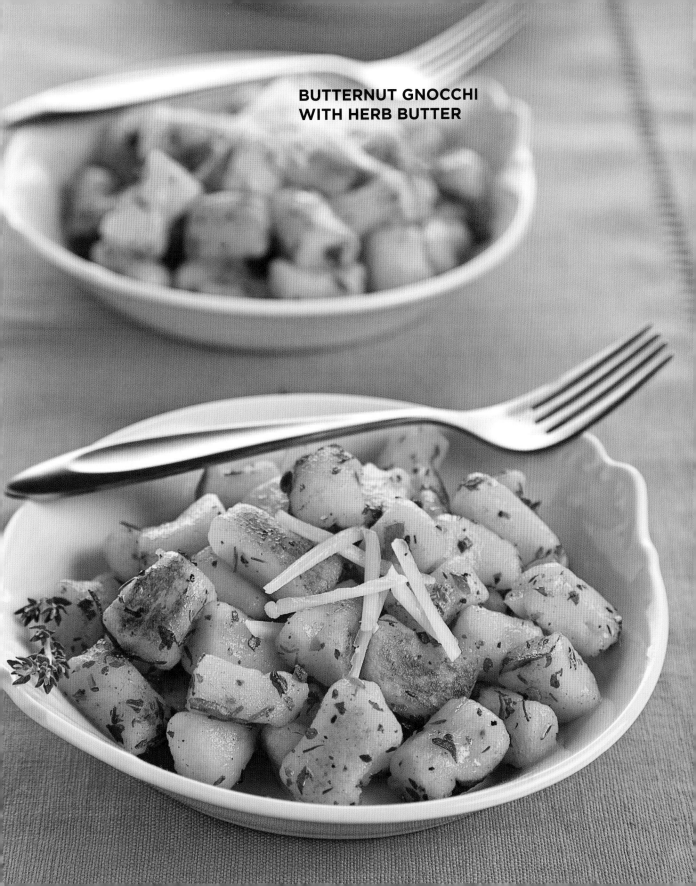

BUTTERNUT GNOCCHI WITH HERB BUTTER

Zucchini Feta Casserole

- 4 medium zucchini
- 1 tablespoon butter
- 2 eggs, beaten
- ½ cup grated Parmesan cheese
- ⅓ cup crumbled feta cheese
- 2 tablespoons chopped fresh parsley
- 1 tablespoon all-purpose flour
- 2 teaspoons chopped fresh marjoram
- Dash hot pepper sauce
- Salt and black pepper

1. Preheat oven to 375°F. Spray 2-quart baking dish with nonstick cooking spray.
2. Grate zucchini; drain well in colander.
3. Melt butter in medium skillet over medium heat. Add zucchini; cook and stir until lightly browned. Remove from heat; stir in eggs, Parmesan, feta, parsley, flour, marjoram, hot pepper sauce, salt and black pepper until well blended. Pour into prepared baking dish.
4. Bake 35 minutes or until hot and bubbly.

Makes 4 servings

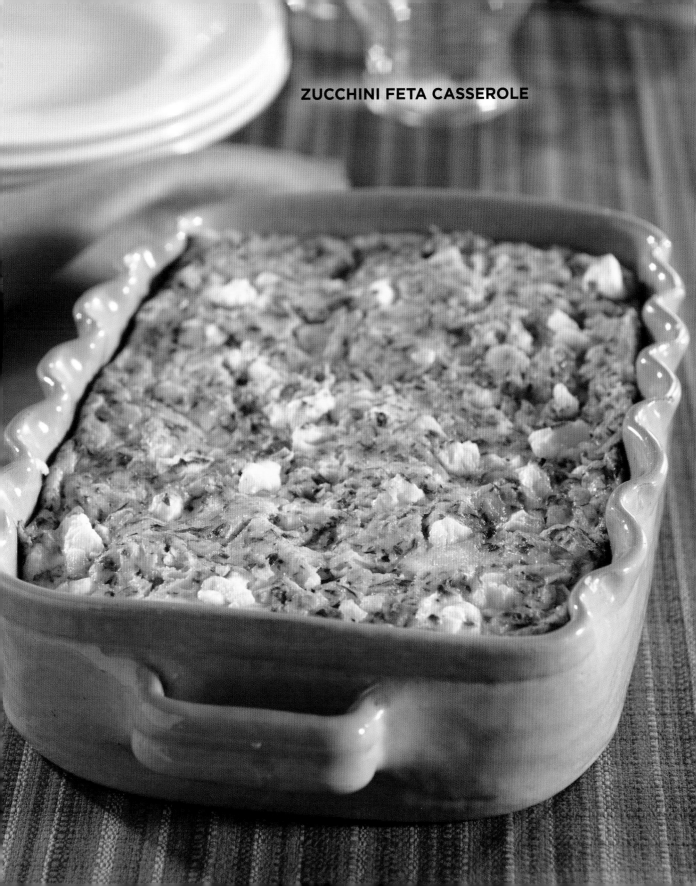

ZUCCHINI FETA CASSEROLE

Spanish Potato Omelet

¼ cup olive oil

¼ cup vegetable oil

1 pound unpeeled red or white potatoes, cut into ⅛-inch slices

½ teaspoon salt, divided

1 small onion, cut in half lengthwise and thinly sliced crosswise

¼ cup chopped green bell pepper

¼ cup chopped red bell pepper

3 eggs

1. Heat olive oil and vegetable oil in large skillet over medium-high heat. Add potatoes; turn several times to coat slices with oil. Sprinkle with ¼ teaspoon salt; cook 6 to 9 minutes or until potatoes are translucent, turning occasionally.

2. Add onion and bell peppers to skillet. Reduce heat to medium; cook 10 minutes or until potatoes are tender, turning occasionally. Drain mixture in colander placed in large bowl; reserve oil. Let potato mixture stand until cool.

3. Beat eggs and remaining ¼ teaspoon salt in separate large bowl. Add potato mixture; gently stir until coated with eggs. Let stand 15 minutes.

4. Heat 2 teaspoons reserved oil in small nonstick skillet over medium-high heat. Spread potato mixture in skillet to form solid layer. Cook until egg mixture on bottom and side of pan is set but top still looks moist. Cover skillet with plate. Flip omelet onto plate, then slide back into skillet. Continue to cook until bottom is lightly browned. Slide omelet onto serving plate. Let stand 30 minutes before serving. Cut into wedges.

Makes 8 servings

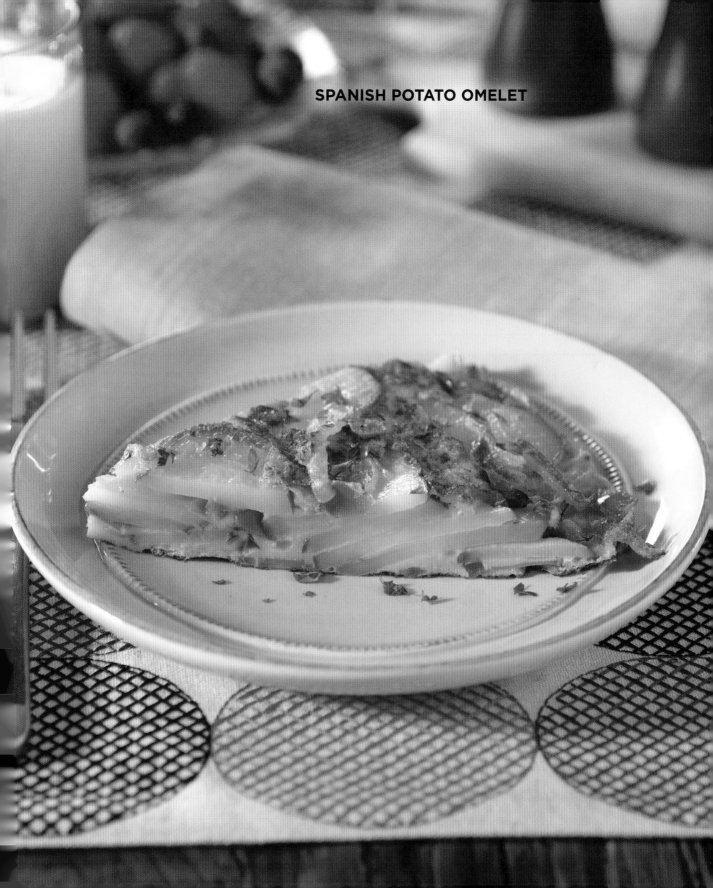

SPANISH POTATO OMELET

Stuffed Chayotes

2 large chayotes

2 tablespoons butter

½ cup chopped onion

1 clove garlic, minced

1 large tomato, peeled, seeded and chopped

2 tablespoons chopped fresh parsley

½ cup cooked whole kernel corn

½ teaspoon salt

⅛ teaspoon black pepper

½ cup (2 ounces) shredded Cheddar cheese

1. Cut chayotes in half lengthwise; retain edible seeds. Place cut sides down on microwavable plate; cook on HIGH 3½ minutes or until tender. When cool enough to handle, remove pulp, leaving ½-inch shells. Coarsely chop pulp and seeds.

2. Preheat oven to 375°F. Spray shallow baking pan with nonstick cooking spray.

3. Melt butter in large skillet over medium heat. Brush inside of chayote shells with half of butter. Add onion and garlic to remaining butter in skillet; cook and stir 3 minutes or until onion is tender. Add tomato and parsley; cook 5 minutes or until liquid has evaporated. Stir in corn, salt, pepper and chayote pulp. Place chayote shells in prepared pan. Fill with vegetable mixture; sprinkle with cheese.

4. Bake, uncovered, 15 minutes or until chayotes are heated through and cheese is melted.

Makes 4 servings

Stuffed Summer Squash: Follow directions for Stuffed Chayotes but use 8 large pattypan squash or 8 zucchini (each about 6 inches long) in place of chayotes. Boil whole squash 8 to 10 minutes or until barely tender. After scooping out pulp, turn shells upside down on paper towels to drain before filling. Makes 8 servings.

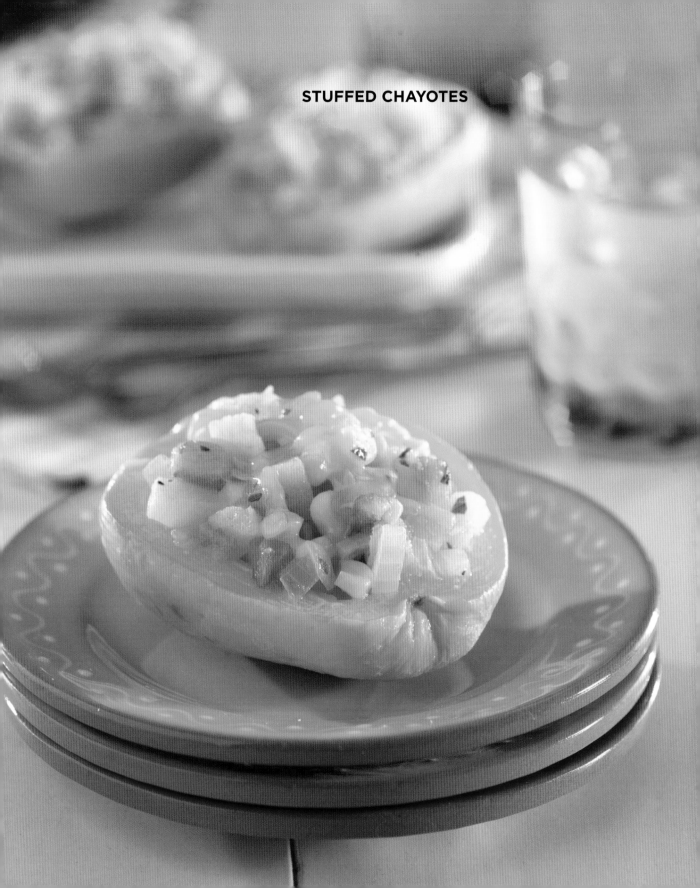

Sweet Potato Gratin

- 3 pounds sweet potatoes (about 5 large)
- ½ cup (1 stick) butter, divided
- ¼ cup plus 2 tablespoons packed brown sugar, divided
- 2 eggs
- ⅔ cup orange juice
- 2 teaspoons ground cinnamon, divided
- ½ teaspoon salt
- ¼ teaspoon ground nutmeg
- ⅓ cup all-purpose flour
- ¼ cup old-fashioned oats
- ⅓ cup chopped pecans or walnuts

1. Preheat oven to 350°F.
2. Bake sweet potatoes 1 hour or until tender. Let stand 5 minutes. Cut sweet potatoes lengthwise into halves; scrape pulp from skins into large bowl.
3. Add ¼ cup butter and 2 tablespoons brown sugar to sweet potato pulp; beat with electric mixer at medium speed until butter is melted. Add eggs, orange juice, 1½ teaspoons cinnamon, salt and nutmeg; beat until smooth. Spoon into six 6-ounce ovenproof baking dishes or ramekins or 1½-quart casserole.
4. Combine flour, oats, remaining ¼ cup brown sugar and ½ teaspoon cinnamon in medium bowl; mix well. Cut in remaining ¼ cup butter with pastry blender or two knives until mixture resembles coarse crumbs. Stir in pecans. Sprinkle evenly over sweet potatoes.
5. Bake 25 to 30 minutes or until heated through. For crispier topping, broil 5 inches from heat source 2 minutes or until golden brown.

Makes 6 to 8 servings

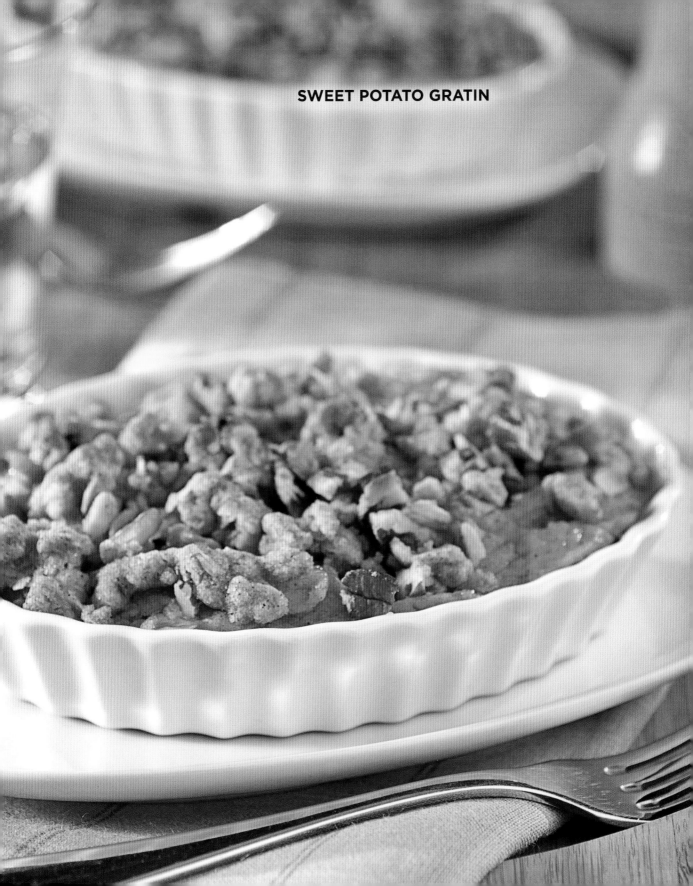

SWEET POTATO GRATIN

Veggie Tostadas

1 tablespoon olive oil

1 cup chopped onion

1 cup chopped celery

2 cloves garlic, minced

1 can (about 15 ounces) red kidney beans, rinsed and drained

1 can (about 15 ounces) Great Northern beans, rinsed and drained

1 can (about 14 ounces) salsa-style diced tomatoes

2 teaspoons mild chili powder

1 teaspoon ground cumin

6 (6-inch) corn tortillas

Optional toppings: chopped fresh cilantro, shredded lettuce, chopped fresh tomatoes, shredded Cheddar cheese and sour cream

1. Heat oil in large skillet over medium heat. Add onion, celery and garlic; cook and stir 8 minutes or until softened. Stir in beans, diced tomatoes, chili powder and cumin. Reduce heat to medium-low; simmer 30 minutes or until thickened, stirring occasionally.

2. Meanwhile, preheat oven to 400°F. Place tortillas in single layer directly on oven rack. Bake 10 to 12 minutes or until crisp.

3. Spread bean mixture evenly over each tortilla; top with cilantro, lettuce, chopped tomatoes, cheese and sour cream, if desired.

Makes 6 servings

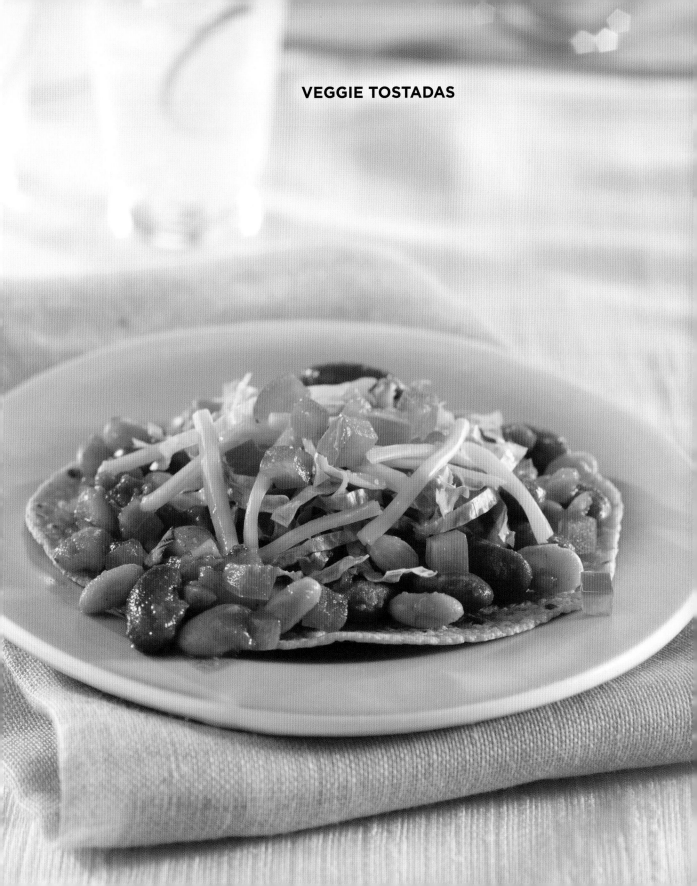

VEGGIE TOSTADAS

Vegetarian Shepherd's Pie

  2 teaspoons olive oil

  1 cup sliced onion

  1 package (16 ounces) white mushrooms, quartered

1¼ teaspoons minced garlic, divided

  1 cup sliced carrots

  1 cup sliced celery

  1 cup frozen green peas

  ¼ cup all-purpose flour

  3 cups vegetable broth

  ¼ teaspoon salt

  ¼ teaspoon dried rosemary

  2 medium russet potatoes, peeled and cubed

  ¼ cup milk

  1 tablespoon butter

  ¼ teaspoon black pepper

     Fresh rosemary sprigs (optional)

1. Heat oil in large saucepan over medium-high heat. Add onion; cook and stir 3 minutes or until just beginning to soften. Add mushrooms; cook and stir 5 minutes or until vegetables are tender. Add 1 teaspoon garlic; cook and stir 1 minute. Add carrots, celery and peas; cook and stir 5 minutes or until crisp-tender.

2. Sprinkle flour over vegetables; cook and stir 2 minutes. Add broth, salt and dried rosemary; bring to a boil. Reduce heat to low; simmer 30 to 35 minutes or until thickened.

3. Meanwhile, place potatoes in medium saucepan; add enough water to cover potatoes. Bring to a boil over high heat. Reduce heat to low; simmer 15 minutes or until tender. Drain potatoes; transfer to medium bowl.

4. Add milk, butter, remaining ¼ teaspoon garlic and pepper to potatoes; beat with electric mixer at low speed until smooth.

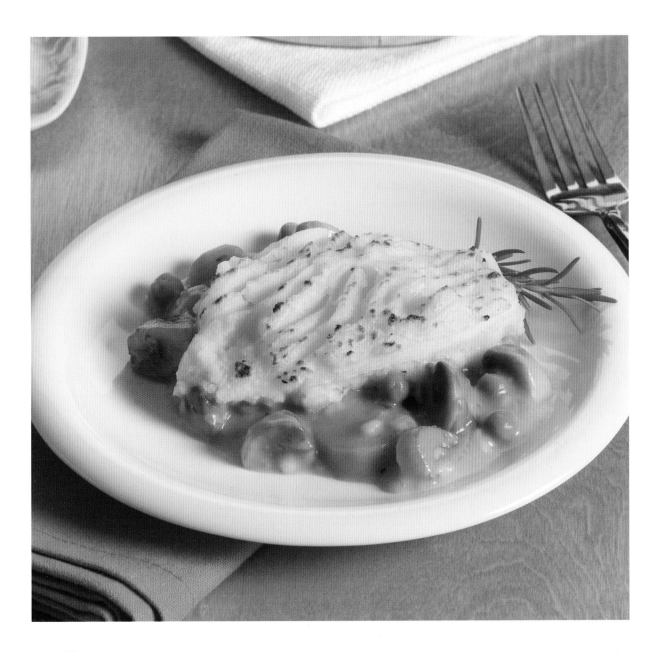

5. Preheat broiler. Pour vegetable mixture into 2-quart casserole; gently spread mashed potatoes over top. Broil 5 minutes or until light golden brown. Garnish with fresh rosemary.

Makes 6 servings

The Vegetarian Cookbook **217**

Skillet Roasted Root Vegetables

- 1 sweet potato, peeled, cut in half lengthwise and cut crosswise into ½-inch slices
- 1 large red onion, cut into 1-inch wedges
- 2 parsnips, cut diagonally into 1-inch slices
- 2 carrots, cut diagonally into 1-inch slices
- 1 turnip, peeled, cut in half and then cut into ½-inch slices
- 2½ tablespoons olive oil
- 1½ tablespoons honey
- 1½ tablespoons balsamic vinegar
- 1 teaspoon coarse salt
- 1 teaspoon dried thyme
- ¼ teaspoon ground red pepper
- ¼ teaspoon black pepper

1. Preheat oven to 400°F.
2. Combine sweet potato, onion, parsnips, carrots, turnip, oil, honey, vinegar, salt, thyme, red pepper and black pepper in large bowl; toss to coat. Spread vegetables in single layer in large cast iron skillet.
3. Roast 1 hour or until vegetables are tender, stirring once halfway through cooking time.

Makes 4 servings

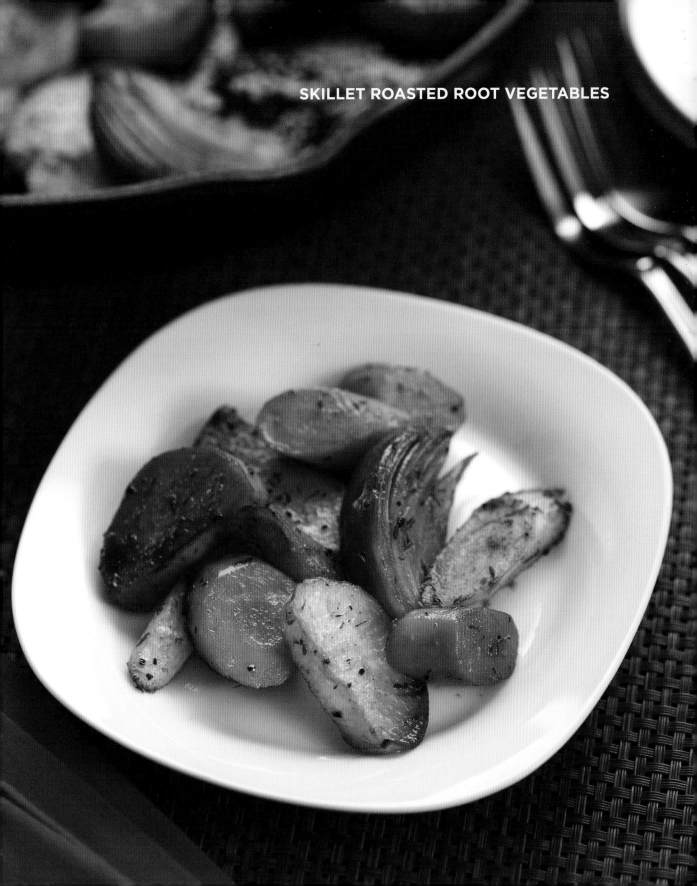

Spaghetti and Vegetable Frittata

- 1 tablespoon olive oil, divided
- 1 package (8 ounces) sliced mushrooms
- 1 cup thinly sliced leeks
- 3 egg whites
- 2 whole eggs
- ⅓ cup milk
- ¼ cup grated Parmesan cheese
- ½ teaspoon salt
- ⅛ teaspoon black pepper
- ⅛ teaspoon ground nutmeg
- 1 package (10 ounces) frozen chopped collard greens, thawed and squeezed dry
- 2 cups cooked whole grain spaghetti
- ½ cup (2 ounces) shredded mozzarella cheese

1. Heat 2 teaspoons oil in large ovenproof skillet over medium-high heat. Add mushrooms and leeks; cook and stir 8 minutes or until lightly browned.

2. Beat egg whites, whole eggs, milk, Parmesan, salt, pepper and nutmeg in large bowl until well blended. Stir in collard greens, spaghetti and mushroom mixture. Preheat broiler.

3. Heat remaining 1 teaspoon oil in same skillet over medium-low heat. Add egg mixture; cover and cook 10 minutes or until top is set.

4. Sprinkle mozzarella over frittata; broil about 5 inches from heat source 3 minutes or until golden brown.

Makes 6 servings

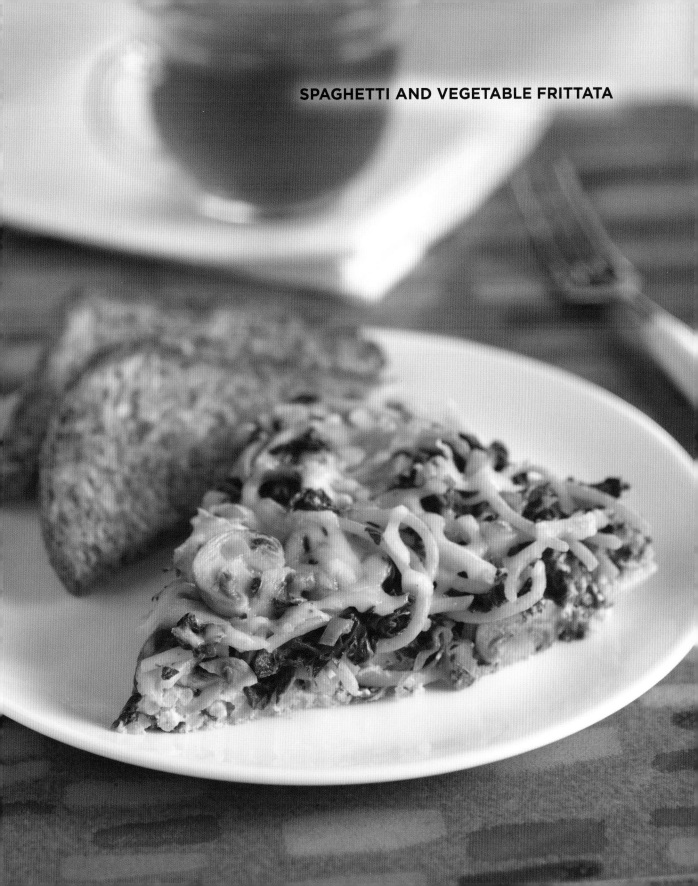

Curried Potatoes, Cauliflower and Peas

1 tablespoon vegetable oil

1 large onion, chopped

2 tablespoons minced fresh ginger

2 cloves garlic, chopped

2 pounds red potatoes, cut into ½-inch-thick slices

1 to 1¼ teaspoons salt

1 teaspoon garam masala*

1 small head cauliflower (about 1¼ pounds), trimmed and broken into florets

1 cup vegetable broth or water

2 ripe plum tomatoes, seeded and chopped

1 cup thawed frozen peas

Hot cooked basmati or long grain rice

Garam masala is a blend of Asian spices available in the spice aisle of many supermarkets. If garam masala is unavailable, substitute ½ teaspoon ground cumin and ½ teaspoon ground coriander seeds.

Slow Cooker Directions

1. Heat oil in large skillet over medium heat. Add onion, ginger and garlic; cook 4 minutes until onion is softened, stirring occasionally.

2. Place potatoes in slow cooker. Combine 1 teaspoon salt and garam masala in small bowl. Sprinkle half of spice mixture over potatoes. Top with onion mixture, then cauliflower. Sprinkle remaining spice mixture over cauliflower. Pour in broth.

3. Cover; cook on HIGH 3½ hours. Gently stir in tomatoes and peas. Cover; cook 30 minutes or until potatoes are tender. Stir gently. Adjust seasoning with additional salt, if desired. Serve over rice.

Makes 6 servings

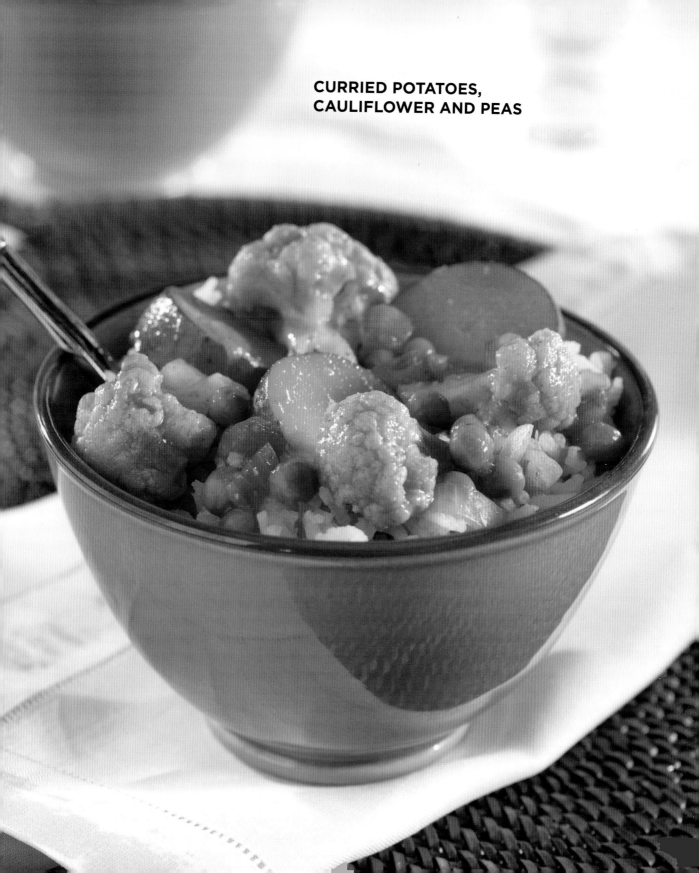

CURRIED POTATOES, CAULIFLOWER AND PEAS

Parsnip Patties

1 pound parsnips, peeled and cut into ¾-inch pieces

¼ cup (½ stick) butter, divided

¼ cup chopped onion

¼ cup all-purpose flour

⅓ cup milk

2 teaspoons chopped fresh chives

Salt and black pepper

¾ cup fresh bread crumbs

2 tablespoons vegetable oil

1. Pour 1 inch water into medium saucepan; bring to a boil over high heat. Add parsnips; cover and cook 10 minutes or until fork-tender. Drain and transfer to large bowl; coarsely mash with fork.

2. Melt 2 tablespoons butter in medium skillet over medium-high heat. Add onion; cook and stir until translucent. Whisk in flour until bubbly and lightly browned. Whisk in milk until thickened. Stir milk mixture into mashed parsnips. Stir in chives; season with salt and pepper.

3. Shape parsnip mixture into four patties. Spread bread crumbs on plate. Dip patties in bread crumbs to coat all sides evenly. Place on waxed paper; refrigerate 2 hours.

4. Heat remaining 2 tablespoons butter and oil in large skillet over medium-high heat until butter is melted and bubbly. Add patties; cook 5 minutes per side or until browned.

Makes 4 servings

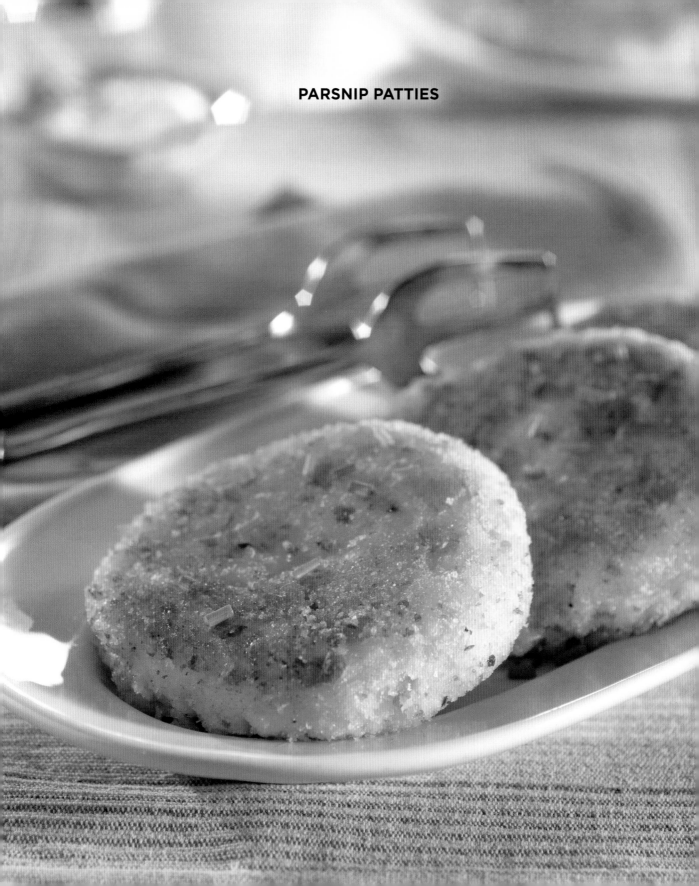

PARSNIP PATTIES

Vegetable Enchiladas

1 tablespoon vegetable oil

2 large poblano peppers or green bell peppers, cut into 2-inch strips

1 large zucchini, cut into 2-inch strips

1 large red onion, sliced

1 cup sliced mushrooms

1 teaspoon ground cumin

1 pound fresh tomatillos (about 8 large), peeled

½ to 1 jalapeño pepper,* minced

1 clove garlic

½ teaspoon salt

1 cup loosely packed fresh cilantro

12 corn tortillas, warmed

2 cups (8 ounces) shredded Mexican cheese blend, divided

*Jalapeño peppers can sting and irritate the skin, so wear rubber gloves when handling peppers and do not touch your eyes.

1. Preheat oven to 400°F. Heat oil in large nonstick skillet over medium heat. Add poblano peppers, zucchini, onion, mushrooms and cumin; cook and stir 8 to 10 minutes or until vegetables are crisp-tender.

2. Meanwhile, place tomatillos in large microwavable bowl; cover with vented plastic wrap. Microwave on HIGH 6 to 7 minutes or until very tender.

3. Combine tomatillos with juice, jalapeño, garlic and salt in food processor or blender; process until smooth. Add cilantro; pulse until combined and cilantro is coarsely chopped.

4. Divide vegetables evenly among tortillas. Spoon heaping tablespoon of cheese in center of each tortilla; roll up to enclose filling. Place in 13×9-inch baking dish. Pour sauce evenly over enchiladas; sprinkle with remaining cheese. Cover with foil.

5. Bake 18 to 20 minutes or until cheese is melted and enchiladas are heated through. Serve immediately.

Makes 6 servings

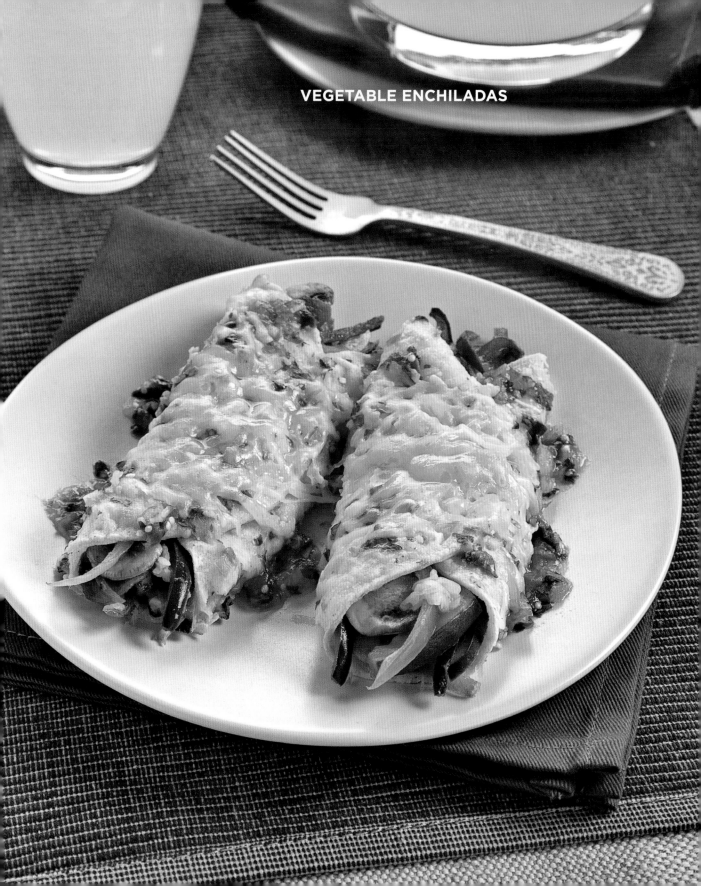

VEGETABLE ENCHILADAS

Potato-Carrot Pancakes

1 pound baking potatoes, peeled (about 3 medium)

1 medium carrot

2 tablespoons minced green onion

1 tablespoon all-purpose flour

1 egg, beaten

½ teaspoon salt

⅛ teaspoon black pepper

2 tablespoons vegetable oil

Green onion strips (optional)

1. Shred potatoes and carrot. Wrap in several sheets of paper towels; squeeze to remove excess moisture.

2. Combine potatoes, carrot, minced green onion, flour, egg, salt and pepper in medium bowl; mix well.

3. Heat oil in large skillet over medium heat. Drop spoonfuls of potato mixture into skillet; flatten to form thin pancakes. Cook 5 minutes per side or until potatoes are tender and pancakes are browned. Garnish with green onion strips.

Makes about 12 pancakes

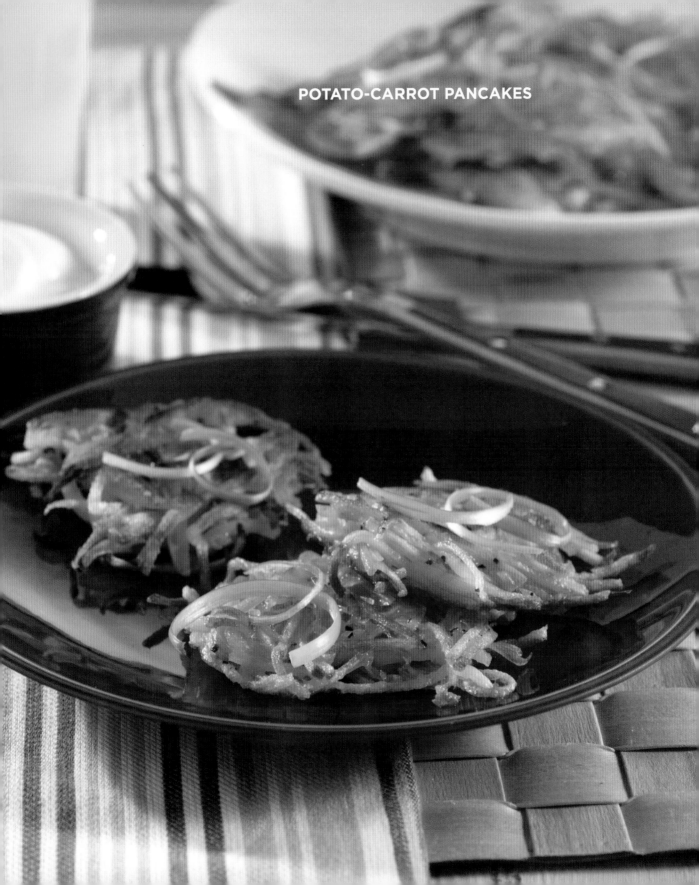

POTATO-CARROT PANCAKES

Spaghetti Squash with Black Beans and Zucchini

1 spaghetti squash (about 2 pounds)

2 medium zucchini, cut lengthwise into ¼-inch-thick slices

2 tablespoons plus 1 teaspoon olive oil, divided

2 cups chopped seeded fresh tomatoes

1 can (about 15 ounces) black beans, rinsed and drained

2 tablespoons chopped fresh basil

2 tablespoons red wine vinegar

1 clove garlic, minced

½ teaspoon salt

1. Prepare grill for direct cooking over medium heat. Pierce spaghetti squash in several places with fork. Place in center of large piece of heavy-duty foil. Bring two long sides of foil together above squash; fold down in series of locked folds, allowing room for heat circulation and expansion. Fold short ends up and over again. Press folds firmly to seal foil packet.

2. Grill squash, covered, 45 minutes to 1 hour or until easily depressed with back of long-handled spoon, turning one quarter turn every 15 minutes. Remove squash from grill; let stand in foil 10 to 15 minutes.

3. Meanwhile, brush both sides of zucchini slices with 1 teaspoon oil. Grill, uncovered, 4 minutes or until tender, turning once. Cut into bite-size pieces.

4. Remove spaghetti squash from foil; cut in half and remove seeds. Separate squash into strands with two forks; place on large serving plate.

5. Combine zucchini, tomatoes, beans and basil in medium bowl; mix well. Whisk remaining 2 tablespoons oil, vinegar, garlic and salt in small bowl until well blended. Add to vegetable mixture; toss gently to coat. Serve over spaghetti squash.

Makes 4 servings

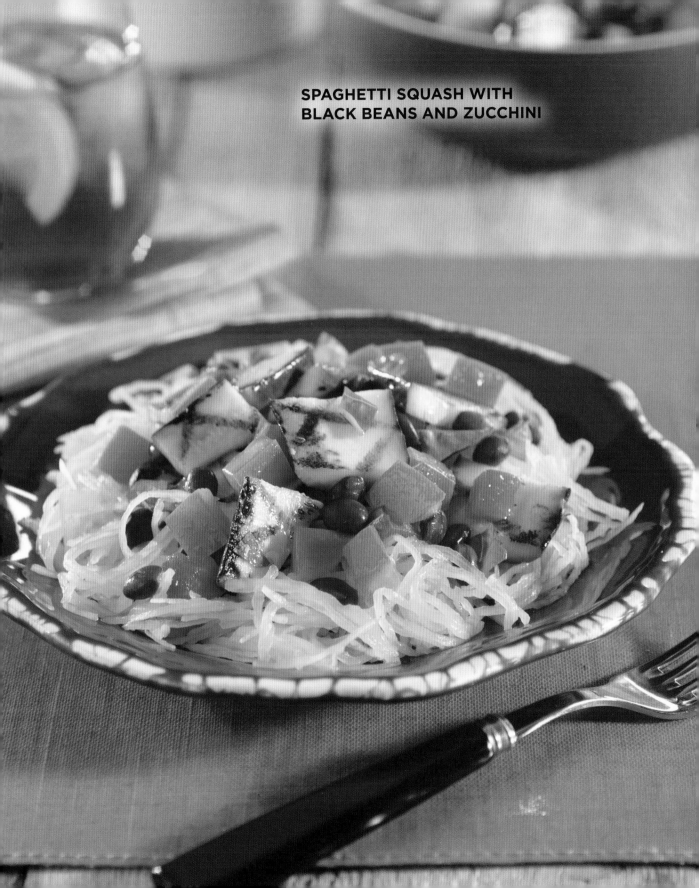

SPAGHETTI SQUASH WITH
BLACK BEANS AND ZUCCHINI

Potato and Leek Gratin

  5 tablespoons butter, divided

  2 large leeks, sliced

  2 tablespoons minced garlic

  2 pounds baking potatoes, peeled (about 4 medium)

  1 cup whipping cream

  1 cup milk

  3 eggs

  2 teaspoons salt

 ¼ teaspoon white pepper

  2 to 3 slices dense day-old white bread, such as French or Italian

 ½ cup grated Parmesan cheese

1. Preheat oven to 375°F. Generously grease shallow 10-cup baking dish with 1 tablespoon butter.

2. Melt 2 tablespoons butter in large skillet over medium heat. Add leeks and garlic; cook and stir 8 to 10 minutes or until leeks are softened. Remove from heat.

3. Cut potatoes crosswise into $\frac{1}{16}$-inch-thick slices. Layer half of potato slices in prepared baking dish; top with half of leek mixture. Repeat layers. Beat cream, milk, eggs, salt and white pepper in medium bowl until well blended; pour evenly over vegetables.

4. Tear bread slices into 1-inch pieces. Place in food processor; process until fine crumbs form. Measure ¾ cup crumbs; place in small bowl. Stir in cheese. Melt remaining 2 tablespoons butter; stir into crumb mixture. Sprinkle crumb mixture over vegetables.

5. Bake about 1 hour 15 minutes or until top is golden brown and potatoes are tender. Let stand 5 to 10 minutes before serving.

Makes 6 to 8 servings

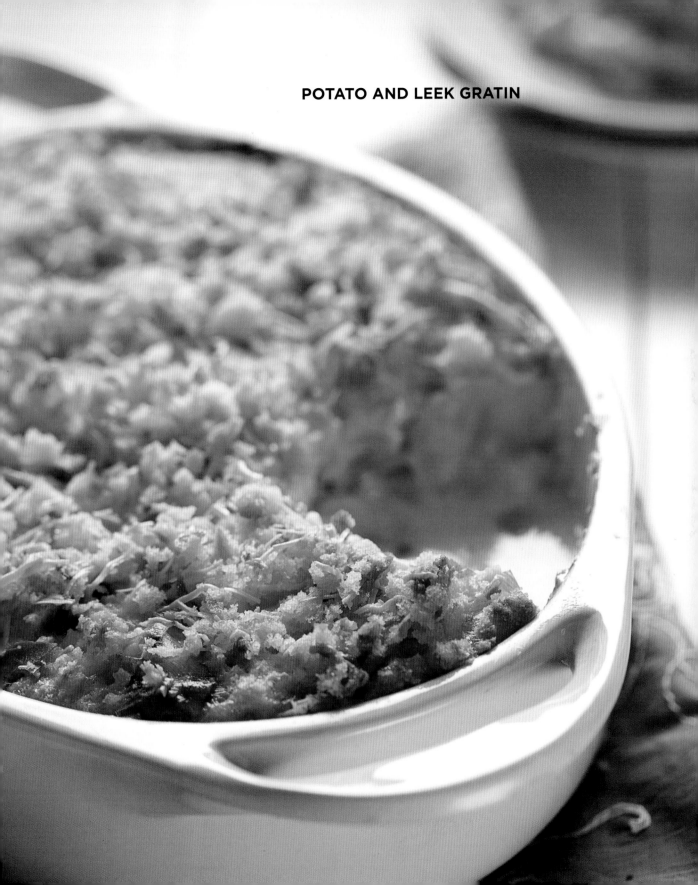

POTATO AND LEEK GRATIN

Layered Butternut Squash Lasagna

- 1 tablespoon olive oil
- 1 small onion, chopped
- 1 package (8 ounces) sliced mushrooms
- 3 cloves garlic, pressed or minced
- 1 can (about 28 ounces) crushed tomatoes, drained, divided
- 1 butternut squash (about 2½ pounds), peeled and cut into ⅛-inch-thick slices
- 1 container (15 ounces) ricotta cheese
- 1 package (8 ounces) shredded mozzarella cheese, divided
- ¼ cup grated Parmesan cheese

1. Heat oven to 350°F. Heat oil in large skillet over medium-high heat. Add onion and mushrooms; cook and stir 5 to 7 minutes. Add garlic; cook and stir 30 seconds. Reduce heat to medium-low; add all but ½ cup tomatoes and simmer 5 minutes.

2. Spread remaining crushed tomatoes on bottom of 13×9-inch baking pan. Layer half of squash over tomatoes. Spread ricotta evenly over squash with back of spoon. Sprinkle with 1 cup mozzarella and half of tomato mixture. Layer with remaining squash, tomato mixture and mozzarella. Sprinkle with Parmesan. Cover with foil sprayed with nonstick cooking spray.

3. Bake 35 minutes. Remove foil; bake 20 to 25 minutes or until squash is tender. Let stand 20 minutes before serving.

Makes 9 servings

Tip: After peeling and seeding the squash, use a mandolin to cut it into thin slices.

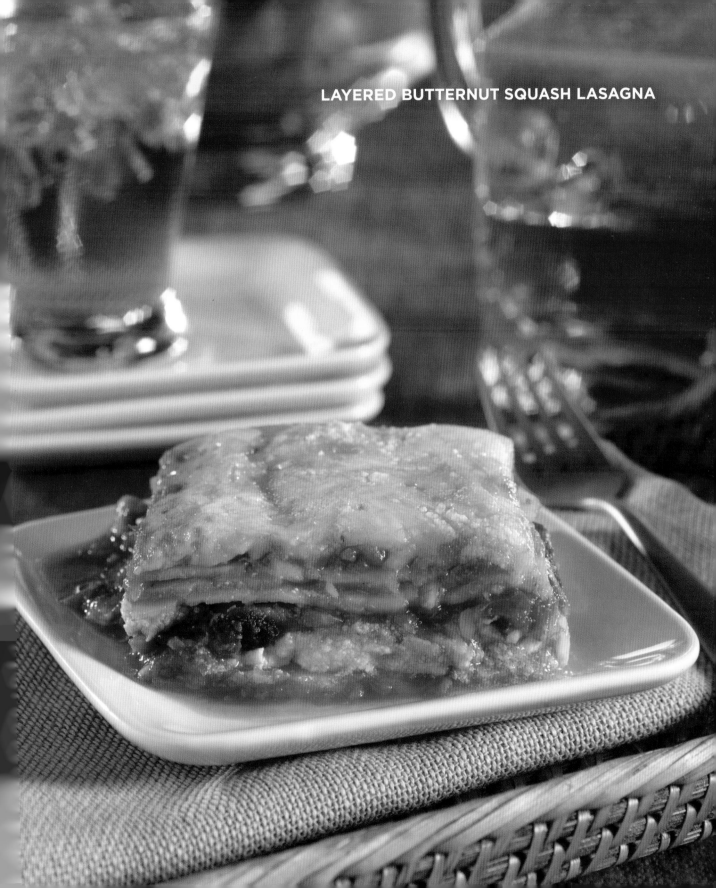

Szechuan Eggplant

1 pound Asian eggplants or regular eggplants, peeled

2 tablespoons peanut or vegetable oil

2 cloves garlic, minced

¼ teaspoon red pepper flakes *or* ½ teaspoon hot chili oil

¼ cup vegetable broth

¼ cup hoisin sauce

3 green onions, cut into 1-inch pieces

Toasted sesame seeds* (optional)

To toast sesame seeds, spread seeds in small skillet. Shake skillet over medium-low heat 3 minutes or until seeds begin to pop and turn golden.

1. Cut eggplants into ½-inch slices; cut each slice into ½×½-inch strips.

2. Heat wok or large skillet over medium-high heat. Add oil; heat until hot. Add eggplants, garlic and red pepper flakes; stir-fry 7 minutes or until eggplants are very tender and browned.

3. Reduce heat to medium. Add broth, hoisin sauce and green onions; cook and stir 2 minutes. Sprinkle with sesame seeds, if desired.

Makes 4 to 6 servings

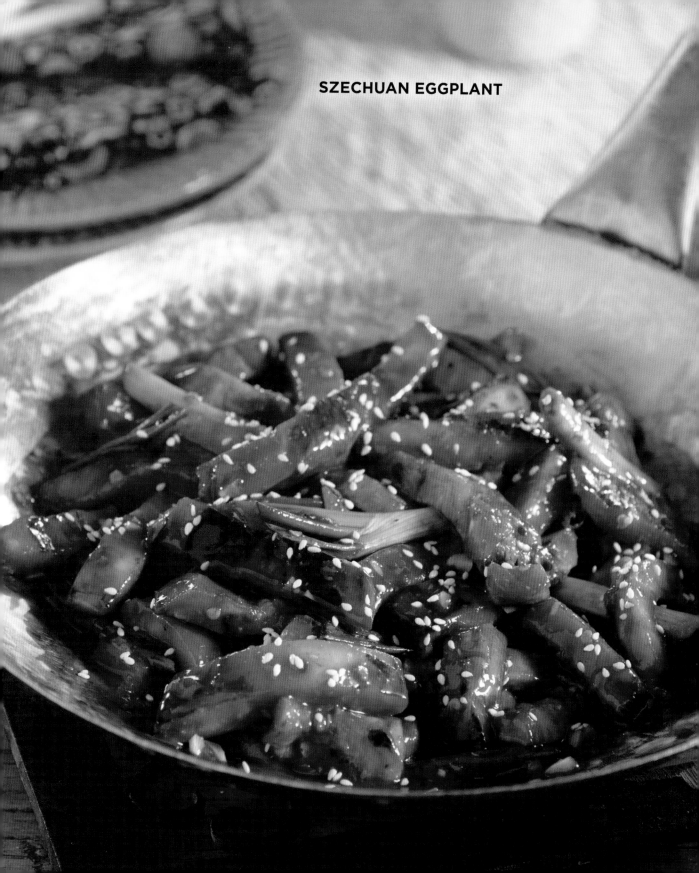

SZECHUAN EGGPLANT

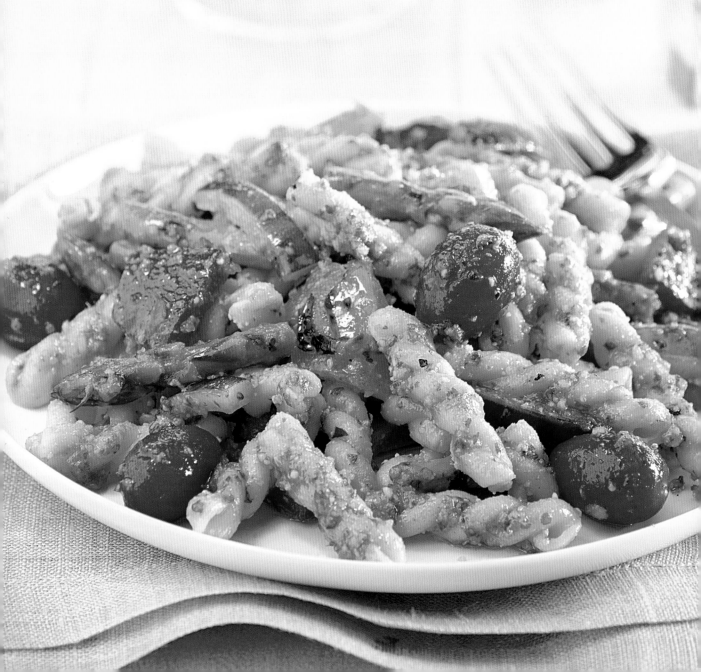

Pasta and Noodles

Gemelli and Grilled Summer Vegetables

- 2 large bell peppers (red and yellow)
- 12 stalks asparagus, trimmed
- 2 slices red onion
- 3 tablespoons plus 1 teaspoon olive oil, divided
- 6 ounces (2¼ cups) uncooked gemelli or rotini pasta
- 2 tablespoons pine nuts
- 1 clove garlic
- 1 cup loosely packed fresh basil leaves
- ¼ cup grated Parmesan cheese
- ¼ teaspoon salt
- ¼ teaspoon black pepper
- 1 cup grape or cherry tomatoes

1. Prepare grill for direct cooking over medium heat. Cut bell peppers in half; remove and discard seeds. Grill bell peppers, skin-side down, covered, 10 to 12 minutes or until skins are blackened. Place peppers in paper or plastic bag; let stand 15 minutes. Remove and discard blackened skins. Cut peppers into large pieces. Place in large bowl.

2. Toss asparagus and onion with 1 teaspoon oil in medium bowl. Grill vegetables, covered, 8 to 10 minutes or until tender, turning once. Cut asparagus into 2-inch pieces; coarsely chop onion. Add to bowl with peppers.

3. Cook pasta according to package directions; drain well and add to vegetables.

4. Combine pine nuts and garlic in food processor; process until coarsely chopped. Add basil; process until finely chopped. With motor running, add remaining 3 tablespoons oil; process until blended. Stir in cheese, salt and black pepper. Add basil mixture and tomatoes to pasta and vegetables; toss to coat. Serve immediately.

Makes 4 servings

Rice Noodles with Broccoli and Tofu

 1 package (14 ounces) firm or extra firm tofu

 1 package (8 to 10 ounces) wide rice noodles

 2 tablespoons peanut oil

 3 medium shallots, sliced

 6 cloves garlic, minced

 1 jalapeño pepper,* minced

 2 teaspoons minced fresh ginger

 3 cups broccoli florets

 ¼ cup soy sauce

 1 to 2 tablespoons fish sauce

   Fresh basil leaves (optional)

*Jalapeño peppers can sting and irritate the skin, so wear rubber gloves when handling peppers and do not touch your eyes.

1. Drain tofu and press between paper towels to remove excess water. Cut tofu into bite-size pieces.

2. Meanwhile, place noodles in medium bowl. Cover with hot water; let stand 15 minutes or until tender. Drain.

3. Heat oil in large skillet or wok over medium-high heat. Add tofu; stir-fry 5 minutes or until lightly browned on all sides. Remove to plate.

4. Add shallots, garlic, jalapeño and ginger to skillet; stir-fry 2 to 3 minutes. Add broccoli; stir-fry 1 minute. Cover and cook 3 minutes or until broccoli is crisp-tender.

5. Add tofu, noodles, soy sauce and fish sauce to skillet; stir-fry 8 minutes or until heated through. Garnish with basil.

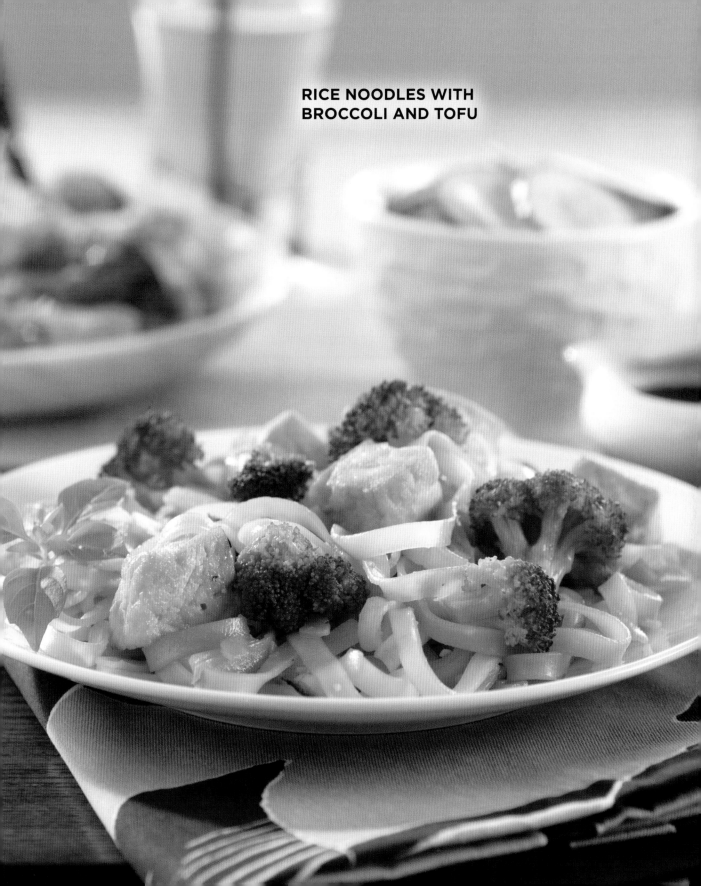

RICE NOODLES WITH BROCCOLI AND TOFU

Pasta with Onions and Goat Cheese

  1 tablespoon olive oil

  3 to 4 cups thinly sliced sweet onions

  ¾ cup (3 ounces) crumbled goat cheese

  ¼ cup milk

  8 ounces uncooked campanelle or farfalle pasta

  1 clove garlic, minced

  2 tablespoons white wine or vegetable broth

1½ teaspoons chopped fresh sage *or* ½ teaspoon dried sage

  ½ teaspoon salt

  ¼ teaspoon black pepper

  2 tablespoons chopped toasted walnuts

1. Heat oil in large skillet over medium heat. Add onions; cook 20 to 25 minutes or until golden brown, stirring occasionally.

2. Combine goat cheese and milk in small bowl; stir until well blended.

3. Cook pasta according to package directions; drain and keep warm.

4. Add garlic to onions in skillet; cook about 3 minutes or until softened. Add wine, sage, salt and pepper; cook until liquid has evaporated. Remove from heat. Add pasta and goat cheese mixture; stir gently until cheese is melted. Sprinkle with walnuts.

Makes 4 to 6 servings

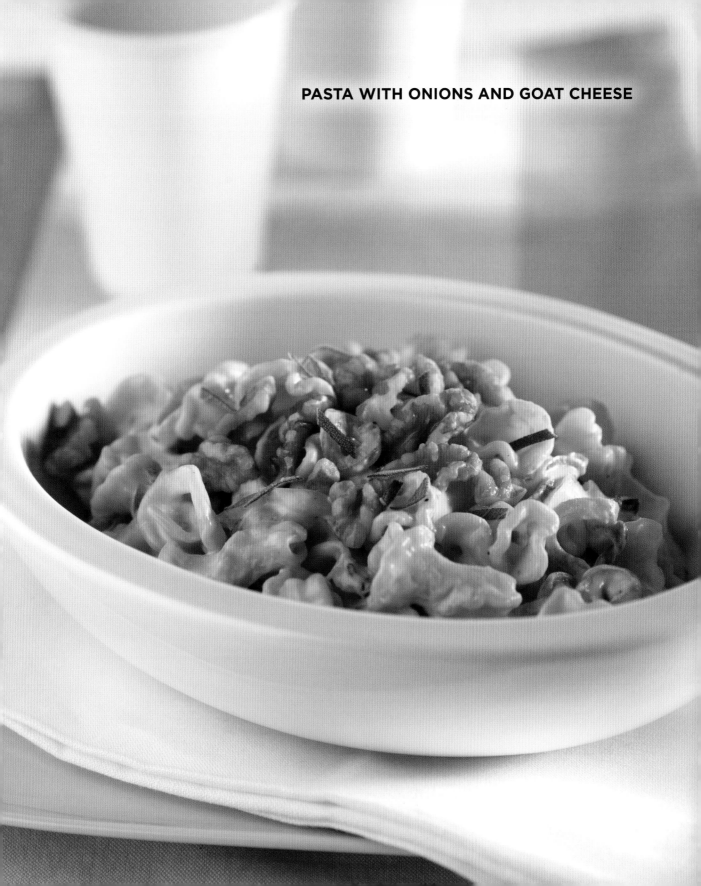

PASTA WITH ONIONS AND GOAT CHEESE

Whole Wheat Spaghetti with Cauliflower and Feta

    3   tablespoons olive oil
    1   onion, chopped
    4   cloves garlic, minced
    1   head cauliflower, cut into bite-size florets
    ⅔   cup white wine or water
    1   teaspoon salt
    ½   teaspoon black pepper
    6   ounces uncooked whole wheat spaghetti
    1   pint grape tomatoes, cut into halves
    ½   cup coarsely chopped walnuts
    ¼   teaspoon red pepper flakes (optional)
    ½   cup (2 ounces) crumbled feta cheese

1. Heat oil in large skillet over medium heat. Add onion; cook and stir 3 minutes or until soft. Add garlic; cook and stir 2 minutes. Add cauliflower; cook and stir 5 minutes. Add wine, salt and pepper; cover and cook about 15 minutes or until cauliflower is crisp-tender.

2. Meanwhile, cook spaghetti according to package directions. Drain pasta, reserving ½ cup cooking water.

3. Add tomatoes, walnuts, red pepper flakes, if desired, and cooking water to skillet; cook 3 minutes or until tomatoes begin to soften.

4. Add spaghetti to skillet; stir to coat with sauce. Sprinkle with cheese.

Makes 4 servings

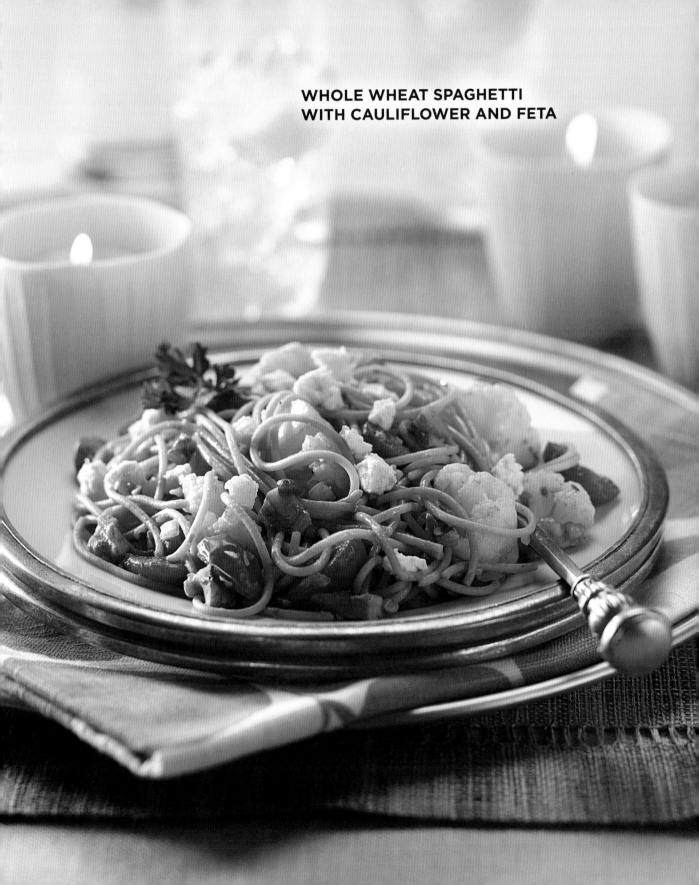

WHOLE WHEAT SPAGHETTI
WITH CAULIFLOWER AND FETA

Zucchini and Mushroom Lasagna with Tofu

- 1 tablespoon olive oil
- 1 cup chopped onion
- 1 package (8 ounces) sliced mushrooms
- 2 small zucchini, thinly sliced
- ½ teaspoon black pepper, divided
- ½ (14-ounce) package soft or firm tofu
- 1 egg
- ¼ teaspoon salt
- 1 jar (26 ounces) spicy red pepper pasta sauce
- 9 uncooked no-boil lasagna noodles
- 2 cups (8 ounces) shredded Italian cheese blend
- ¼ cup grated Parmesan cheese

1. Preheat oven to 350°F. Spray 9-inch square baking dish with nonstick cooking spray.

2. Heat oil in large skillet over medium-high heat. Add onion; cook and stir 2 minutes. Add mushrooms, zucchini and ¼ teaspoon pepper; cook about 8 minutes or until vegetables are crisp-tender.

3. Meanwhile, combine tofu, egg, salt and remaining ¼ teaspoon pepper in medium bowl; stir until well blended and smooth.

4. Spread ½ cup pasta sauce over bottom of prepared baking dish. Top with 3 noodles, one third of vegetable mixture, one third of tofu mixture, one third of remaining pasta sauce and one third of Italian cheese blend. Repeat layers twice. Cover with foil.

5. Bake 1 hour. Remove foil; sprinkle with Parmesan. Bake, uncovered, 15 minutes or until cheese is browned. Let stand 15 minutes before serving.

Makes 4 to 6 servings

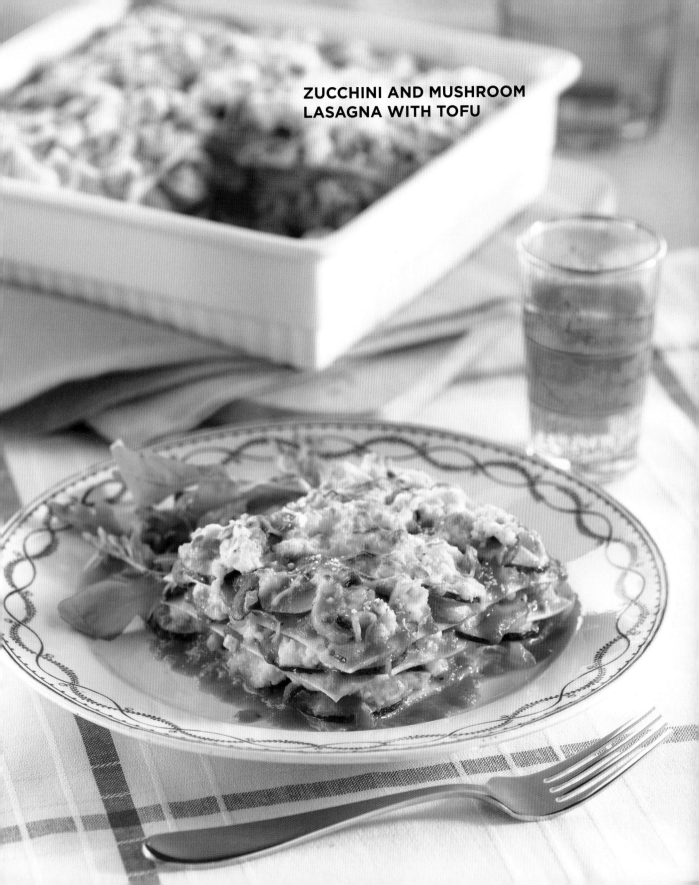
ZUCCHINI AND MUSHROOM
LASAGNA WITH TOFU

Vegetable Lo Mein

8 ounces uncooked Chinese egg noodles or thin spaghetti

2 eggs

1 green onion, thinly sliced

1 teaspoon peanut oil

1 tablespoon dark sesame oil

4 ounces shiitake mushrooms, tough stems discarded, caps sliced *or* 1 package (4 ounces) sliced exotic mushrooms

2 cups thinly sliced bok choy (leaves and stems)

1 small red or yellow bell pepper, cut into strips

½ cup reduced-sodium vegetable broth

¼ cup reduced-sodium teriyaki sauce

Chopped peanuts (optional)

Chopped fresh cilantro (optional)

1. Cook noodles according to package directions; drain.

2. Beat eggs in small bowl until foamy. Stir in green onion. Heat peanut oil in large nonstick skillet over medium heat. Add egg mixture; cook, without stirring, 2 to 3 minutes or until bottom is set. Gently turn; cook 1 minute or until bottom is set. Remove to cutting board; set aside.

3. Heat sesame oil in same skillet over medium-high heat. Add mushrooms, bok choy and bell pepper; cook and stir 4 to 5 minutes or until vegetables are tender. Add broth and teriyaki sauce; cook 2 minutes. Remove to large bowl. Add noodles; toss to coat.

4. Cut egg pancake into strips; add to noodle mixture. Gently toss to combine. Sprinkle with peanuts and cilantro, if desired.

Makes 4 servings

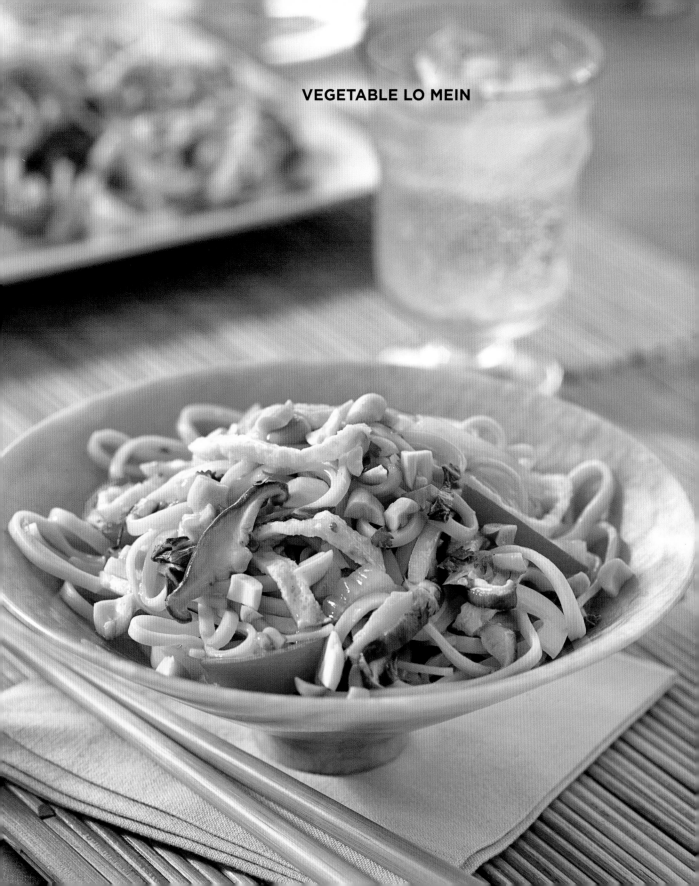

VEGETABLE LO MEIN

Tofu Rigatoni Casserole

3 cups uncooked rigatoni pasta

4 cups loosely packed baby spinach

1 cup soft tofu

1 egg

¼ teaspoon salt

¼ teaspoon black pepper

¼ teaspoon ground nutmeg (optional)

1 can (about 14 ounces) diced tomatoes with basil, garlic and oregano

1 can (about 14 ounces) quartered artichoke hearts, drained and chopped

2 cups (8 ounces) shredded Italian cheese blend, divided

1. Preheat oven to 350°F. Spray 11×7-inch baking dish with nonstick cooking spray.

2. Cook pasta in large saucepan according to package directions. Stir in spinach in bunches during last 2 minutes of cooking. Drain pasta and spinach; return to saucepan.

3. Meanwhile, combine tofu, egg, salt, pepper and nutmeg, if desired, in medium bowl; stir until well blended. Add to pasta mixture in saucepan; mix gently. Add tomatoes, artichokes and 1½ cups cheese; mix well. Spoon into prepared baking dish.

4. Bake 20 minutes. Top with remaining ½ cup cheese; bake 10 minutes or until cheese is browned.

Makes 6 servings

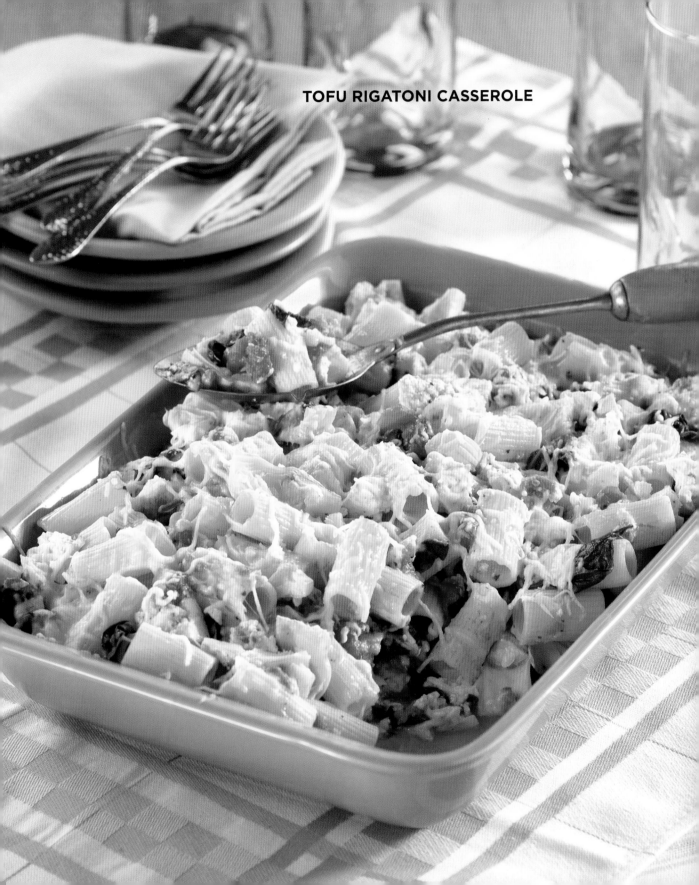

TOFU RIGATONI CASSEROLE

Creamy Fettuccine with Asparagus and Lima Beans

    8 ounces uncooked fettuccine
    2 tablespoons butter
    2 cups fresh asparagus pieces (about 1-inch pieces)
    1 cup frozen lima beans, thawed
    ¼ teaspoon black pepper
    ½ cup vegetable broth
    1 cup half-and-half or whipping cream
    1 cup grated Parmesan cheese

1. Cook fettuccine according to package directions; drain and keep warm.

2. Meanwhile, melt butter in large skillet over medium-high heat. Add asparagus, lima beans and pepper; cook and stir 3 minutes. Add broth; cook 3 minutes. Add half-and-half; cook 3 to 4 minutes or until vegetables are tender, stirring occasionally.

3. Add vegetable mixture and cheese to fettuccine; toss to coat. Serve immediately.

Makes 4 servings

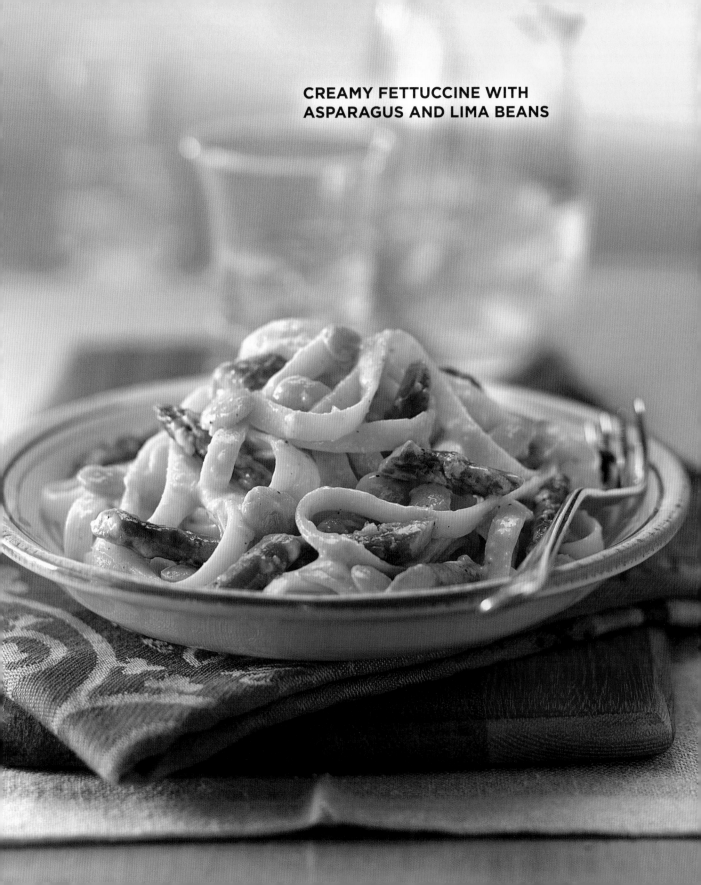

CREAMY FETTUCCINE WITH ASPARAGUS AND LIMA BEANS

Cauliflower Mac and Gouda

1 package (about 16 ounces) bowtie pasta

4 cups milk

2 cloves garlic, peeled and smashed

¼ cup (½ stick) plus 3 tablespoons butter, divided

5 tablespoons all-purpose flour

1 pound Gouda cheese, shredded

1 teaspoon dry mustard

⅛ teaspoon smoked paprika or paprika

Salt and black pepper

1 head cauliflower, cored and cut into florets

1 cup panko bread crumbs

1. Cook pasta according to package directions until almost tender. Drain pasta, reserving pasta water; keep warm. Return water to a boil.

2. Bring milk and garlic to a boil in small saucepan over high heat. Discard garlic; keep milk warm over low heat.

3. Melt ¼ cup butter in large saucepan over medium heat; whisk in flour. Cook 1 minute, whisking constantly. Gradually add warm milk, whisking constantly. Bring to a boil. Reduce heat to low; cook 10 minutes or until thickened, whisking frequently. Remove from heat.

4. Add cheese, mustard and paprika to milk mixture; whisk until melted. Season with salt and pepper. Keep warm.

5. Preheat broiler. Add cauliflower to boiling pasta water; cook 3 to 5 minutes or just until tender. Drain cauliflower; add to sauce mixture with pasta and toss to coat. Spoon into 10 to 12 ramekins or 13×9-inch baking dish.

6. Melt remaining 3 tablespoons butter in small saucepan over medium heat. Add panko; cook and stir just until moistened. Sprinkle over pasta mixture. Broil 2 minutes or until golden brown.

Makes 10 to 12 side-dish or 6 to 8 main-dish servings

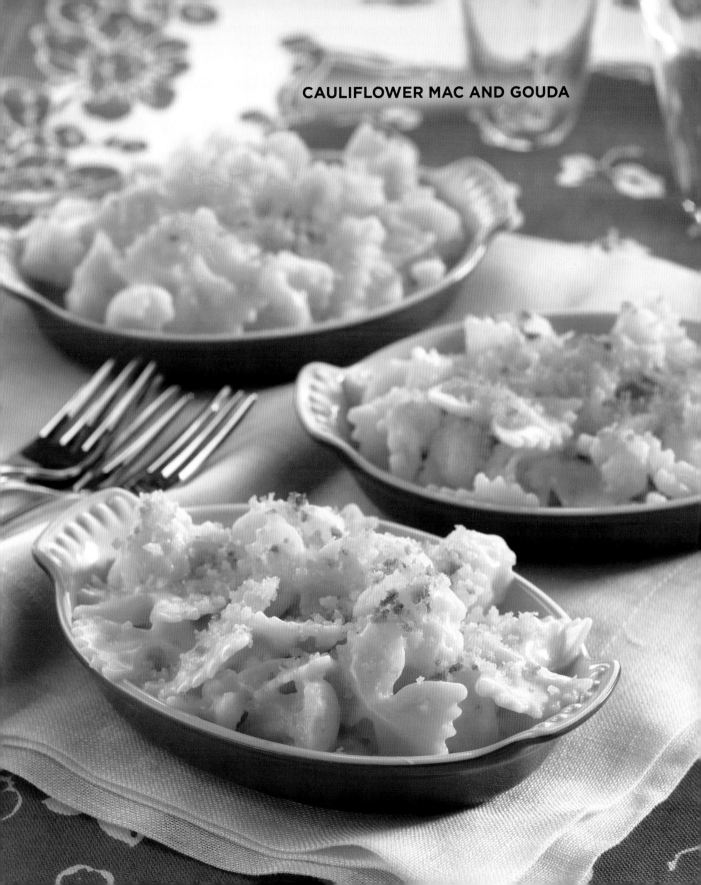

CAULIFLOWER MAC AND GOUDA

Szechuan Cold Noodles

8 ounces vermicelli pasta, broken in half, or Chinese egg noodles

3 tablespoons rice vinegar

3 tablespoons soy sauce

2 tablespoons peanut or vegetable oil

1 clove garlic, minced

1 teaspoon minced fresh ginger

1 teaspoon dark sesame oil (optional)

½ teaspoon crushed Szechuan peppercorns or red pepper flakes

½ cup coarsely chopped fresh cilantro

¼ cup chopped peanuts

1. Cook pasta according to package directions; drain.
2. Whisk vinegar, soy sauce, peanut oil, garlic, ginger, sesame oil, if desired, and peppercorns in large bowl until well blended. Add hot pasta; toss to coat. Sprinkle with cilantro and peanuts. Serve at room temperature or chilled.

Makes 4 servings

Szechuan Vegetable Noodles: Add 1 cup chopped peeled cucumber, ½ cup chopped red bell pepper, ½ cup sliced green onions and an additional 1 tablespoon soy sauce.

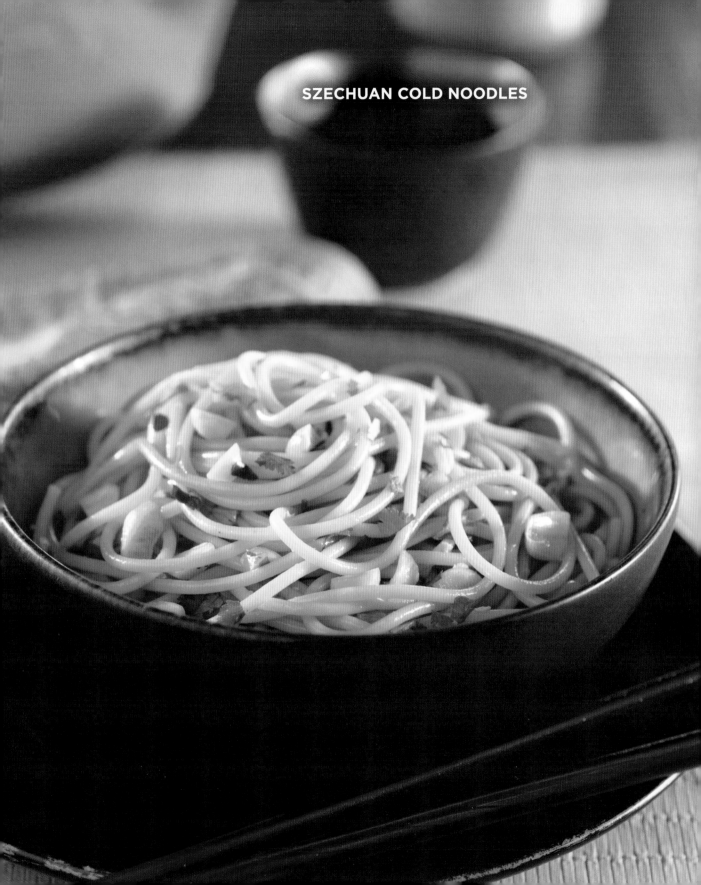

SZECHUAN COLD NOODLES

Pesto Lasagna

1 package (16 ounces) uncooked lasagna noodles

3 tablespoons olive oil

1½ cups chopped onions

3 cloves garlic, finely chopped

3 packages (10 ounces each) frozen chopped spinach, thawed and squeezed dry

Salt and black pepper

3 cups (24 ounces) ricotta cheese

1½ cups pesto sauce

¾ cup grated Parmesan cheese

½ cup pine nuts, toasted*

4 cups (16 ounces) shredded mozzarella cheese

Roasted red pepper strips (optional)

To toast pine nuts, cook in small heavy skillet over medium heat 1 to 2 minutes or until lightly browned, stirring frequently. Immediately remove from skillet; cool before using.

1. Preheat oven to 350°F. Spray 13×9-inch baking dish or lasagna pan with nonstick cooking spray. Partially cook lasagna noodles according to package directions.

2. Heat oil in large skillet over medium-high heat. Add onions and garlic; cook and stir 5 minutes or until translucent. Add spinach; cook and stir about 5 minutes. Season with salt and black pepper. Transfer to large bowl.

3. Add ricotta, pesto, Parmesan and pine nuts to spinach mixture; mix well.

4. Place five lasagna noodles, slightly overlapping, in prepared baking dish. Top with one third of ricotta mixture and one third of mozzarella. Repeat layers twice.

5. Bake about 35 minutes or until hot and bubbly. Garnish with roasted pepper strips.

Makes 8 servings

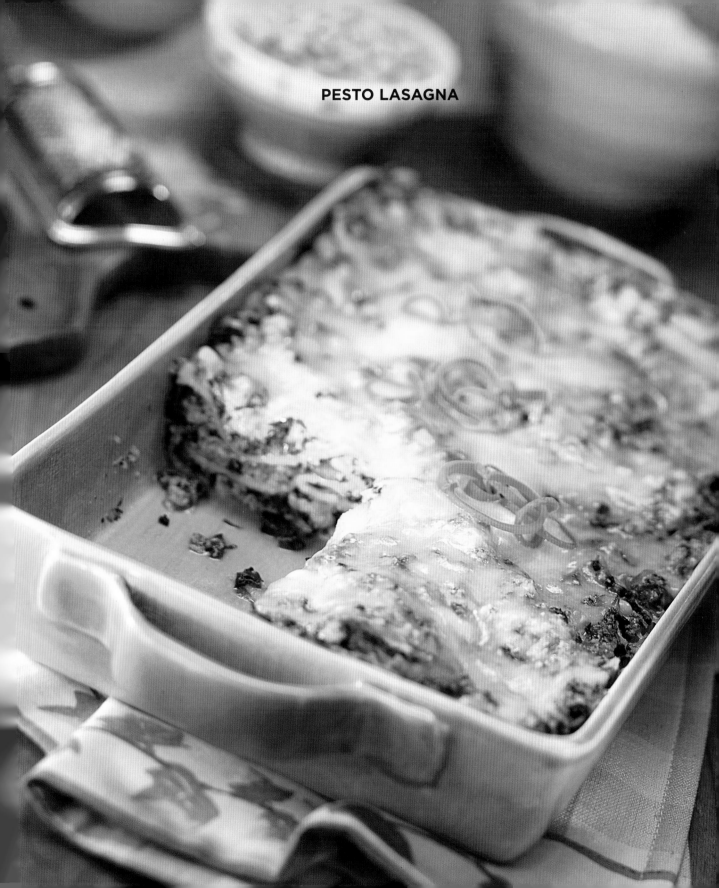

PESTO LASAGNA

Vegetarian Rice Noodles

½ cup soy sauce

⅓ cup sugar

¼ cup lime juice

2 fresh red Thai chiles *or* 1 large jalapeño pepper,* finely chopped

8 ounces thin rice noodles (rice vermicelli)

¼ cup vegetable oil

8 ounces firm tofu, drained and cut into triangles

1 jicama (8 ounces), peeled and chopped *or* 1 can (8 ounces) sliced water chestnuts, drained

2 medium sweet potatoes (1 pound), peeled and cut into ¼-inch-thick slices

2 large leeks, cut into ¼-inch-thick slices

¼ cup chopped unsalted dry-roasted peanuts

2 tablespoons chopped fresh mint

2 tablespoons chopped fresh cilantro

Chile peppers can sting and irritate the skin, so wear rubber gloves when handling peppers and do not touch your eyes.

1. Whisk soy sauce, sugar, lime juice and chiles in small bowl until well blended; set aside.

2. Place rice noodles in medium bowl. Cover with hot water; let stand 15 minutes or until soft. Drain well; cut into 3-inch lengths.

3. Meanwhile, heat oil in large skillet over medium-high heat. Add tofu; stir-fry 4 minutes per side or until golden. Remove with slotted spatula to paper towel-lined baking sheet.

4. Add jicama to skillet; stir-fry 5 minutes or until lightly browned. Remove to baking sheet. Stir-fry sweet potatoes in batches until tender and browned; remove to baking sheet. Add leeks; stir-fry 1 minute. Remove to baking sheet.

5. Stir soy sauce mixture; add to skillet. Cook until sugar dissolves. Add noodles; toss to coat. Gently stir in tofu, vegetables, peanuts, mint and cilantro.

Makes 4 servings

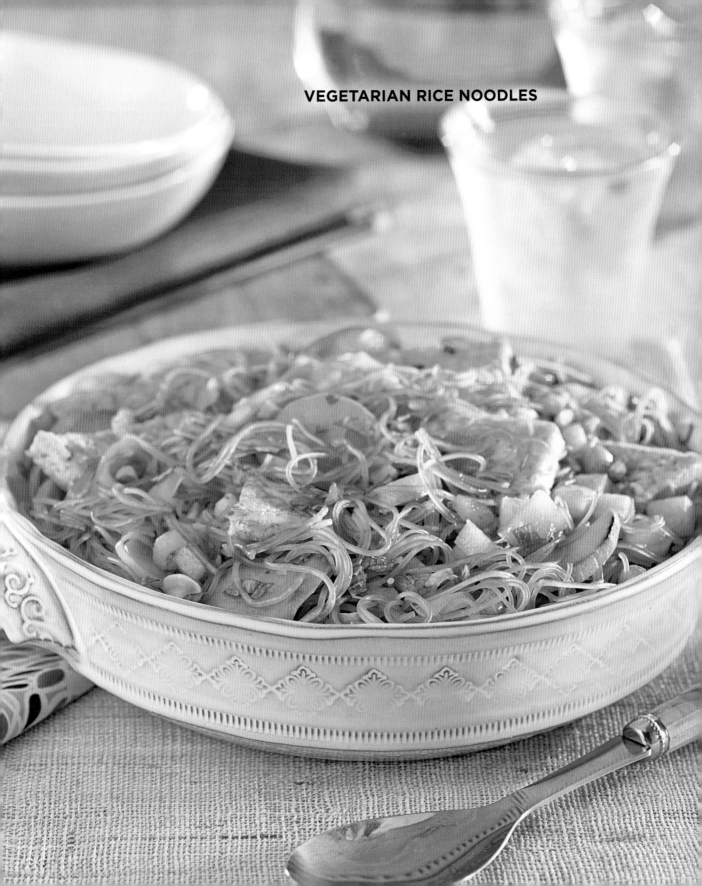

VEGETARIAN RICE NOODLES

Spinach Gnocchi

2 packages (10 ounces each) frozen chopped spinach

1 cup ricotta cheese

2 eggs

⅓ cup grated Parmesan cheese

3 tablespoons all-purpose flour

½ teaspoon salt

⅛ teaspoon black pepper

⅛ teaspoon ground nutmeg

Marinara sauce

Shaved Parmesan cheese

1. Cook spinach according to package directions. Drain well; set aside until cool enough to handle. Squeeze spinach dry; place in medium bowl. Stir in ricotta, eggs, grated Parmesan, flour, salt, pepper and nutmeg until well blended. Cover and refrigerate 1 hour.

2. Line baking sheet with parchment paper. Press heaping tablespoonful of spinach mixture between spoon and your hand to form oval gnocchi; place on prepared baking sheet. Repeat with remaining spinach mixture. Freeze gnocchi 30 minutes.

3. Bring large pot of salted water to a boil over medium-high heat. Drop 8 to 12 gnocchi into boiling water; cook, uncovered, about 2½ minutes or until gnocchi float to surface. Remove gnocchi with slotted spoon; drain on paper towel-lined plate. Return water to a boil; repeat with remaining gnocchi.

4. Serve gnocchi with marinara sauce and shaved Parmesan.

Makes 4 to 6 servings (about 32 gnocchi)

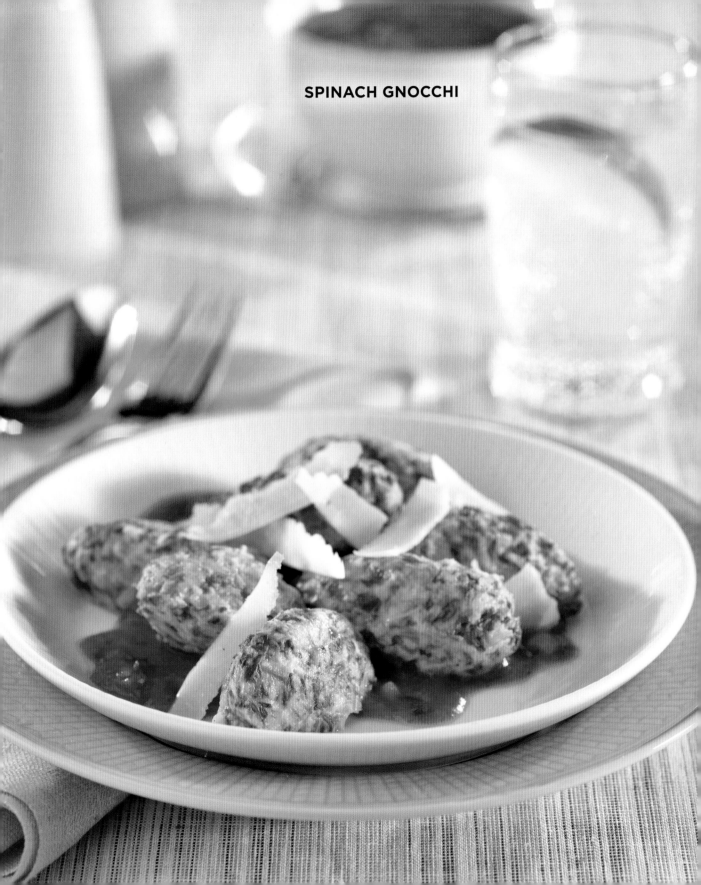

SPINACH GNOCCHI

Peanut-Sauced Pasta

⅓ cup vegetable broth

3 tablespoons creamy peanut butter

2 tablespoons seasoned rice vinegar

2 tablespoons reduced-sodium soy sauce

½ teaspoon red pepper flakes

9 ounces uncooked multigrain linguine

1½ pounds fresh asparagus, cut into 1-inch pieces (4 cups)

⅓ cup dry-roasted peanuts, chopped

1. Whisk broth, peanut butter, vinegar, soy sauce and red pepper flakes in small saucepan until smooth. Cook over low heat until heated through, stirring frequently. Keep warm.

2. Cook linguine according to package directions. Add asparagus to saucepan during last 5 minutes of cooking. Drain linguine and asparagus; toss with peanut sauce. Sprinkle with peanuts.

Makes 6 servings

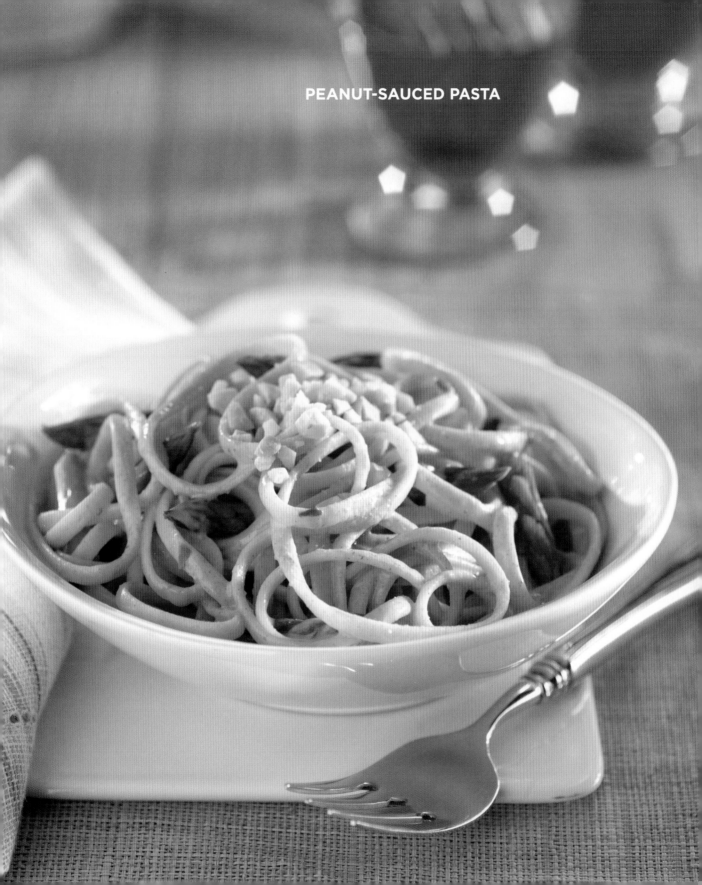

PEANUT-SAUCED PASTA

Eggplant Rigatoni

8 ounces uncooked whole wheat rigatoni pasta

2 tablespoons olive oil, divided

2 medium eggplant, peeled and cut into 1-inch cubes

Salt and black pepper

½ cup (2 ounces) herb goat cheese

1. Cook pasta according to package directions. Drain pasta, reserving 1 cup cooking water.

2. Meanwhile, heat 1 tablespoon oil in large nonstick skillet over medium heat. Add eggplant; cook and stir 20 minutes or until eggplant is soft and golden brown.

3. Add reserved cooking water to eggplant; mix well. Add pasta, remaining 1 tablespoon oil, salt and pepper; mix gently. Cook until heated through. Stir in cheese.

Makes 4 to 6 servings

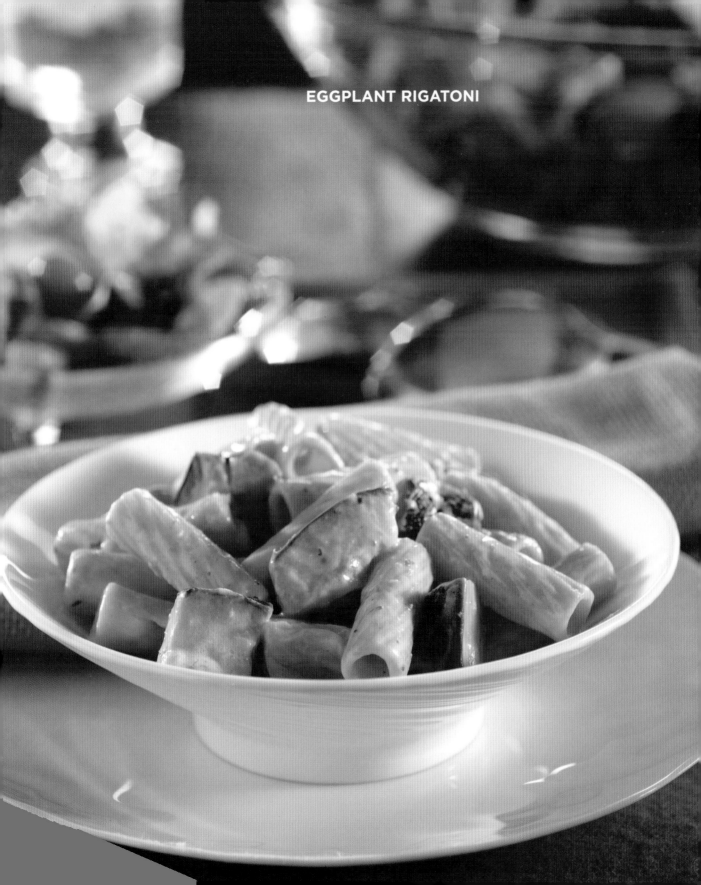

EGGPLANT RIGATONI

Spaghetti Aglio e Olio

 8 ounces uncooked spaghetti or thin spaghetti

⅓ cup plus 1 tablespoon olive oil, divided

 1 cup fresh Italian or French bread crumbs*

 4 cloves garlic, very thinly sliced

¾ teaspoon salt

½ teaspoon red pepper flakes

½ cup chopped fresh Italian parsley

¾ cup shredded Parmesan cheese, divided

To make fresh bread crumbs, tear 2 ounces bread into pieces; process in food processor until coarse crumbs form.

1. Cook spaghetti according to package directions; Drain pasta, reserving ½ cup cooking water.

2. Meanwhile, heat 1 tablespoon oil in large skillet over medium heat. Add bread crumbs; cook 4 to 5 minutes or until golden brown, stirring frequently. Transfer to small bowl.

3. Add remaining ⅓ cup oil, garlic, salt and red pepper flakes to same skillet; cook about 3 minutes or until edges of garlic are just beginning to brown.

4. Add spaghetti and parsley to skillet; toss to coat. Add some of reserved cooking water to moisten spaghetti, if desired. Stir in bread crumbs and ½ cup cheese. Top with remaining ¼ cup cheese.

Makes 4 servings

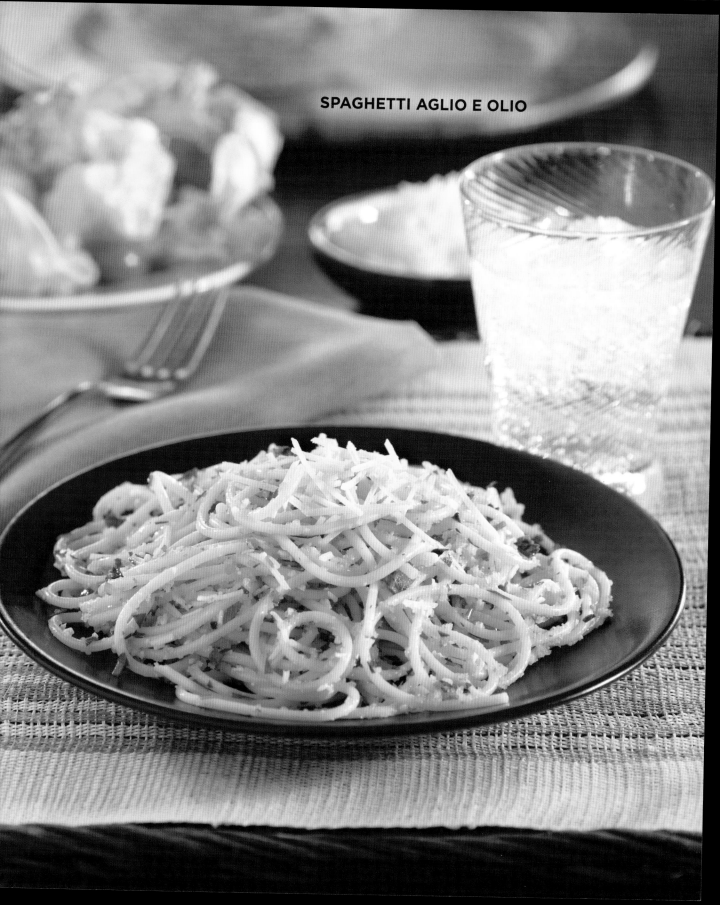

SPAGHETTI AGLIO E OLIO

Vegan Mushroom Gratin

- 4 tablespoons dairy-free margarine, divided
- 1 small onion, minced
- 8 ounces (about 2½ cups) sliced cremini mushrooms
- 2 cloves garlic, minced
- 4 cups cooked elbow macaroni, rotini or other pasta
- 2 tablespoons all-purpose flour
- 1 cup unsweetened soymilk
- ½ teaspoon salt
- ½ teaspoon black pepper
- ½ teaspoon dry mustard
- ½ cup fresh bread crumbs
- 1 tablespoon extra virgin olive oil

1. Preheat oven to 350°F. Spray shallow baking dish with nonstick cooking spray. Melt 2 tablespoons margarine in large skillet over medium-high heat. Add onion; cook and stir 2 minutes. Add mushrooms and garlic; cook and stir 6 to 8 minutes or until vegetables soften. Remove from heat; stir in macaroni.

2. Melt remaining 2 tablespoons margarine in medium saucepan over low heat. Whisk in flour; cook and stir 2 minutes without browning. Add soymilk; bring to a boil over medium-high heat, whisking constantly. Reduce heat to maintain a simmer. Add salt, pepper and mustard; cook 5 to 7 minutes or until sauce thickens, whisking constantly.

3. Pour sauce over mushroom mixture in skillet; stir to coat. Spoon into prepared baking dish. Top with bread crumbs; drizzle with oil. Cover with foil.

4. Bake 15 minutes. Remove foil; bake 10 minutes or until bubbly and browned.

Makes 8 servings

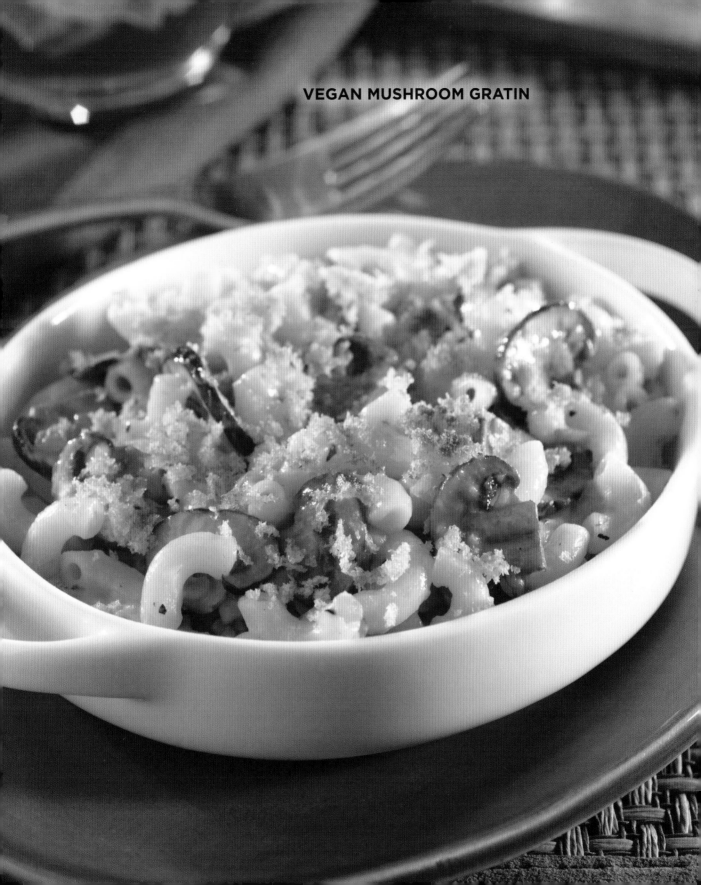
VEGAN MUSHROOM GRATIN

Cheesy Spinach Bake

    8 ounces uncooked spinach fettuccine
    1 tablespoon vegetable oil
 1½ cups sliced mushrooms
    2 green onions, finely chopped
    1 teaspoon garlic, minced
    1 package (10 ounces) frozen spinach, thawed and squeezed dry*
    2 tablespoons water
    1 container (15 ounces) ricotta cheese
   ¾ cup whipping cream
    1 egg
   ½ teaspoon ground nutmeg
   ½ teaspoon black pepper
   ½ cup (2 ounces) shredded Swiss cheese

*Or substitute 10 ounces coarsely chopped fresh baby spinach.

1. Preheat oven to 350°F. Spray 1½-quart baking dish with nonstick cooking spray. Cook fettuccine according to package directions; drain.

2. Heat oil in medium skillet over medium heat. Add mushrooms, green onions and garlic; cook and stir until mushrooms are softened. Stir in spinach and water; cover and cook about 3 minutes or until spinach is wilted.

3. Combine ricotta, cream, egg, nutmeg and pepper in large bowl; mix well. Gently stir in noodles and vegetables until blended. Spread noodle mixture in prepared baking dish; sprinkle with Swiss cheese.

4. Bake 25 to 30 minutes or until knife inserted halfway into center comes out clean.

Makes 6 servings

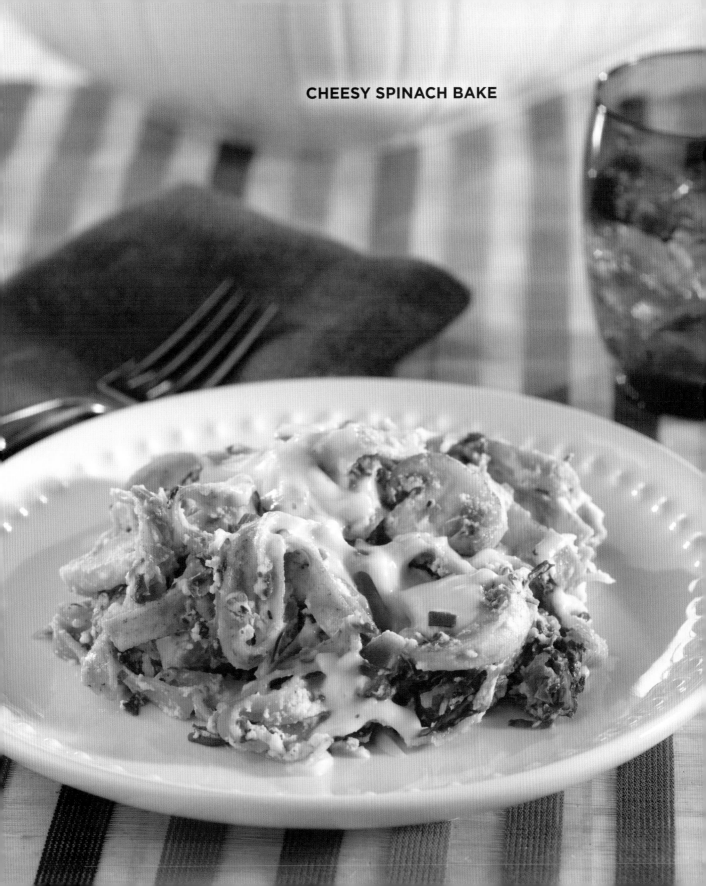

CHEESY SPINACH BAKE

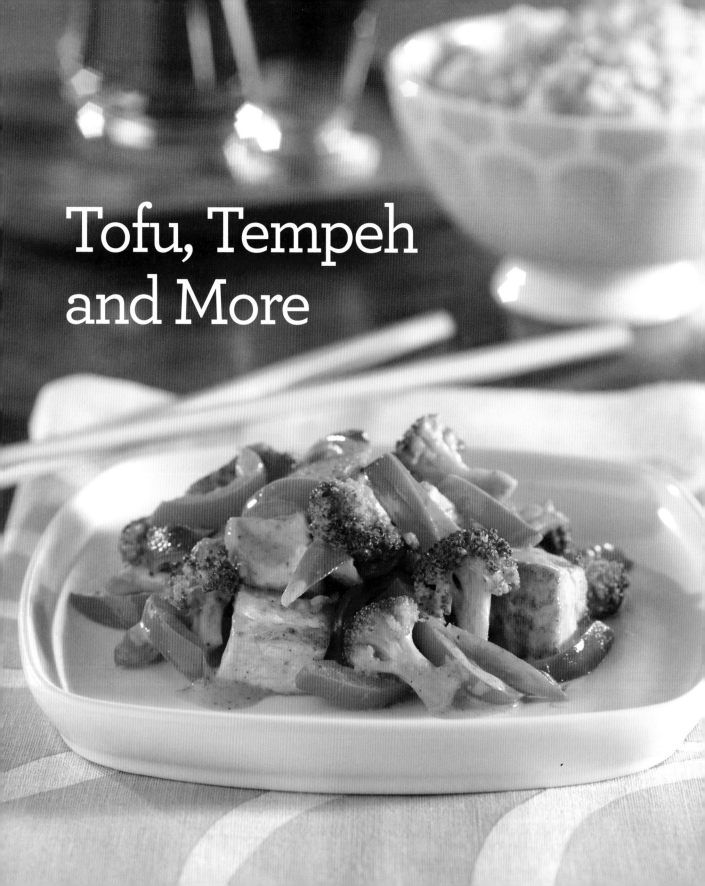

Tofu, Tempeh and More

Tofu, Vegetable and Curry Stir-Fry

1 package (about 14 ounces) extra firm tofu, cut into ¾-inch cubes

¾ cup reduced-fat coconut milk

2 tablespoons fresh lime juice

1 tablespoon curry powder

2 teaspoons dark sesame oil, divided

4 cups broccoli florets (1½-inch pieces)

2 medium red bell peppers, cut into short thin strips

1 medium red onion, cut into thin wedges

¼ teaspoon salt

Hot cooked brown rice (optional)

1. Press tofu cubes between layers of paper towels to remove excess moisture. Combine coconut milk, lime juice and curry powder in medium bowl; mix well.

2. Heat 1 teaspoon oil in large nonstick skillet over medium heat. Add tofu; cook 10 minutes or until lightly browned on all sides, turning frequently. Remove to plate.

3. Heat remaining 1 teaspoon oil in same skillet over high heat. Add broccoli, bell pepper and onion; stir-fry about 5 minutes or until vegetables are crisp-tender. Stir in tofu and coconut milk mixture; cook and stir until mixture comes to a boil. Stir in salt. Serve immediately with rice, if desired.

Makes 4 servings

Teriyaki Tempeh with Pineapple

- 1 cup water
- 1 package (8 ounces) unseasoned tempeh, cut in half crosswise
- 1 to 1½ cups pineapple teriyaki sauce
- 1 cup uncooked rice
- ½ cup matchstick-size carrots
- ½ cup snow peas
- ½ cup matchstick-size red bell pepper strips
- 4 fresh pineapple rings

1. Combine water and tempeh in large deep skillet; bring to a boil over high heat. Reduce heat to low; simmer 10 minutes. Drain water; add 1 cup teriyaki sauce to tempeh in skillet. Bring to a simmer over medium heat; simmer 10 minutes, turning tempeh occasionally. Drain and reserve teriyaki sauce; add additional sauce, if necessary, to make ½ cup.

2. Meanwhile, cook rice according to package directions. Heat reserved teriyaki sauce in wok or large nonstick skillet over medium-high heat. Add carrots, snow peas and bell pepper; cook and stir 4 to 6 minutes or until crisp-tender. Add rice; stir to combine. Add additional teriyaki sauce, if desired.

3. Prepare grill for direct cooking over medium-high heat. Grill tempeh and pineapple rings 10 minutes, turning once. Cut tempeh in half; serve with rice and pineapple.

Makes 4 servings

Island Tempeh Sandwiches: Omit rice and vegetables. Serve tempeh and pineapple on soft rolls with arugula, additional teriyaki sauce and mayonnaise, if desired.

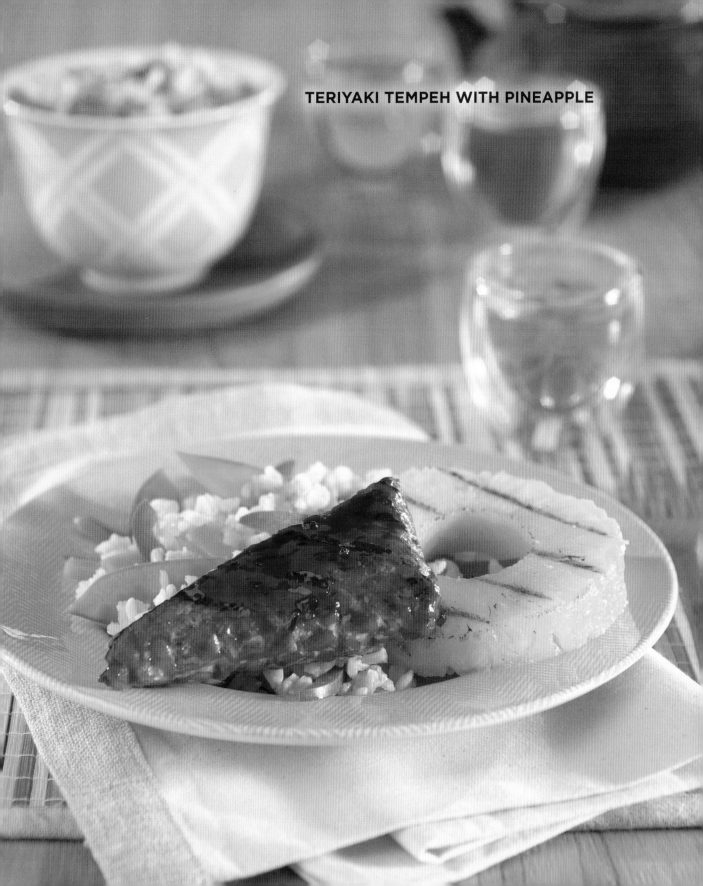

TERIYAKI TEMPEH WITH PINEAPPLE

Fried Tofu with Asian Vegetables

1 package (14 ounces) firm tofu

½ cup reduced-sodium soy sauce, divided

1 cup all-purpose flour

¾ teaspoon salt, divided

⅛ teaspoon black pepper

Vegetable oil for frying

2 packages (16 ounces each) frozen mixed Asian vegetables*

3 tablespoons water

1 teaspoon cornstarch

3 tablespoons plum sauce

2 tablespoons lemon juice

2 teaspoons sugar

1 teaspoon minced fresh ginger

⅛ to ¼ teaspoon red pepper flakes

*Frozen vegetables do not need to be thawed before cooking.

1. Drain tofu; cut into ¾-inch cubes. Combine tofu and ¼ cup soy sauce in shallow bowl; let stand 5 minutes. Combine flour, ½ teaspoon salt and black pepper on plate. Gently toss tofu cubes, a few at a time, with flour mixture to coat.

2. Heat 1½ inches oil in Dutch oven or wok. Test heat by dropping 1 tofu cube into oil; it should brown in 1 minute. Fry tofu cubes in small batches until browned. Remove from oil with slotted spoon; drain on paper towel-lined plate.

3. Pour off all but 1 tablespoon oil from Dutch oven. Add frozen vegetables and remaining ¼ teaspoon salt; cook over medium-high heat about 6 minutes or until vegetables are heated through, stirring occasionally. Increase heat to high to evaporate any remaining liquid. Transfer to large bowl; keep warm.

4. Stir water into cornstarch in small bowl until well blended. Combine cornstarch mixture, remaining ¼ cup soy sauce, plum sauce, lemon juice, sugar, ginger and red pepper flakes in small saucepan; cook and stir over low heat 1 to 2 minutes or until sauce is slightly thickened. Add sauce and tofu to vegetables; toss gently to coat.

Makes 6 servings

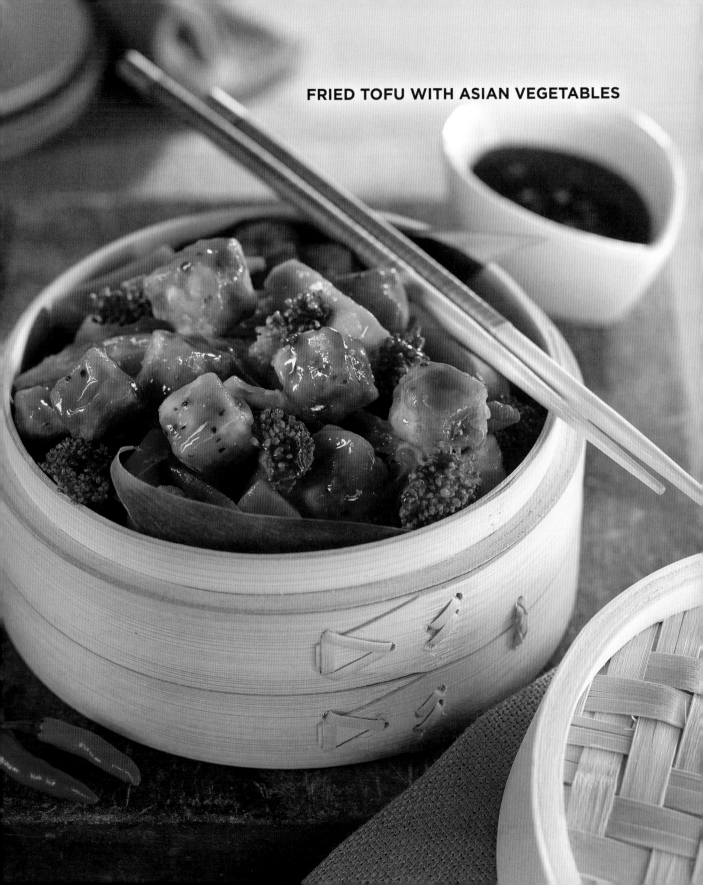

FRIED TOFU WITH ASIAN VEGETABLES

Grilled Seitan and Vegetable Skewers

  1 package (8 ounces) seitan, cubed

 ½ cup barbecue sauce, divided

  1 red bell pepper, cut into 12 pieces

  1 green bell pepper, cut into 12 pieces

 12 mushrooms

  1 zucchini, cut into 12 pieces

1. Place seitan in medium bowl. Add ¼ cup barbecue sauce; mix well. Marinate in refrigerator 30 minutes. Soak four bamboo skewers in water 20 minutes.

2. Prepare grill for direct cooking over medium-high heat. Oil grid. Thread seitan, bell peppers, mushrooms and zucchini onto skewers.

3. Grill skewers, covered, 8 minutes or until seitan is hot and glazed with sauce, brushing with some of remaining sauce and turning occasionally.

Makes 4 servings

Barbecue Tofu

  1 package (14 ounces) extra firm tofu

  1 bottle (18 ounces) barbecue sauce

  4 to 6 pieces frozen Texas toast, prepared according to package directions

    Coleslaw

1. Place tofu on paper towel-lined plate; cover with another paper towel. Place weighted saucepan or baking dish on top of tofu. Let stand 15 minutes to drain. Cut tofu into eight equal slices.

2. Spread half of barbecue sauce in large skillet; arrange tofu slices over sauce in single layer. Cover with remaining sauce. Cover and cook over medium heat about 10 minutes or until heated through, carefully turning tofu after 5 minutes.

3. Serve tofu over Texas toast. Drizzle with sauce; serve with coleslaw.

Makes 4 to 6 servings

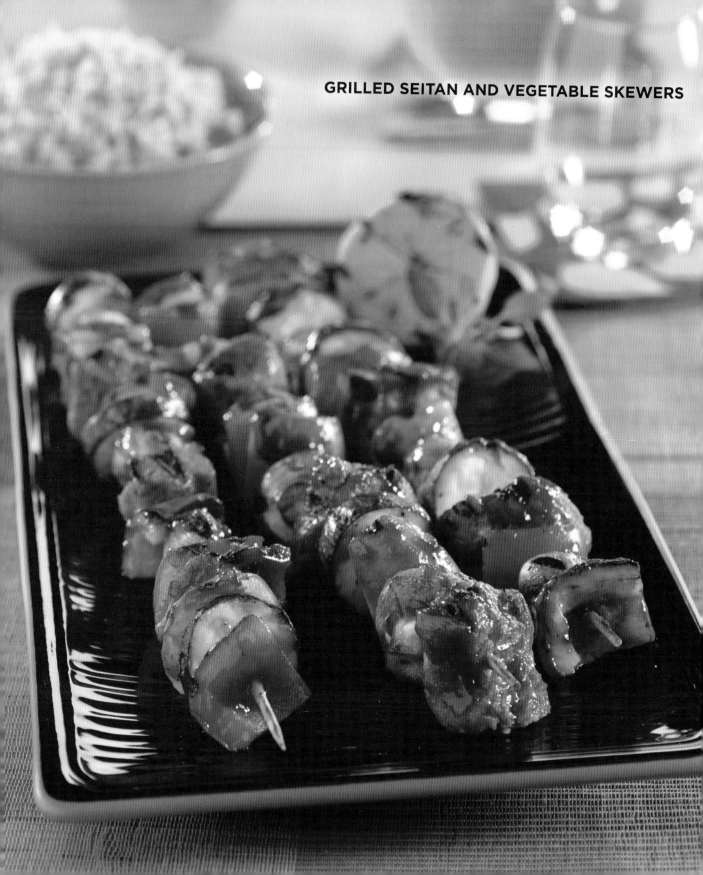

Sesame Ginger-Glazed Tofu with Rice

1 package (14 ounces) extra firm tofu

1 cup sesame ginger stir-fry sauce, divided

1 cup uncooked long grain rice

4 medium carrots, chopped (about 1 cup)

4 ounces snow peas, halved (about 1 cup)

1. Cut tofu in half crosswise; cut each half diagonally into two triangles. Place tofu triangles on cutting board between layers of paper towels. Place another cutting board on top to press moisture out of tofu. Let stand about 15 minutes.

2. Spread ½ cup stir-fry sauce in baking dish. Place tofu in sauce; marinate at room temperature 30 minutes, turning after 15 minutes.

3. Meanwhile, cook rice according to package directions; keep warm.

4. Spray indoor grill pan with nonstick cooking spray; heat over medium-high heat. Grill tofu 6 to 8 minutes or until lightly browned, turning after 4 minutes.

5. Pour remaining ½ cup stir-fry sauce into large nonstick skillet; heat over medium-high heat. Add carrots and snow peas; cook and stir 4 to 6 minutes or until crisp-tender. Add rice; stir to combine.

6. Divide rice mixture among four plates; top with tofu.

Makes 4 servings

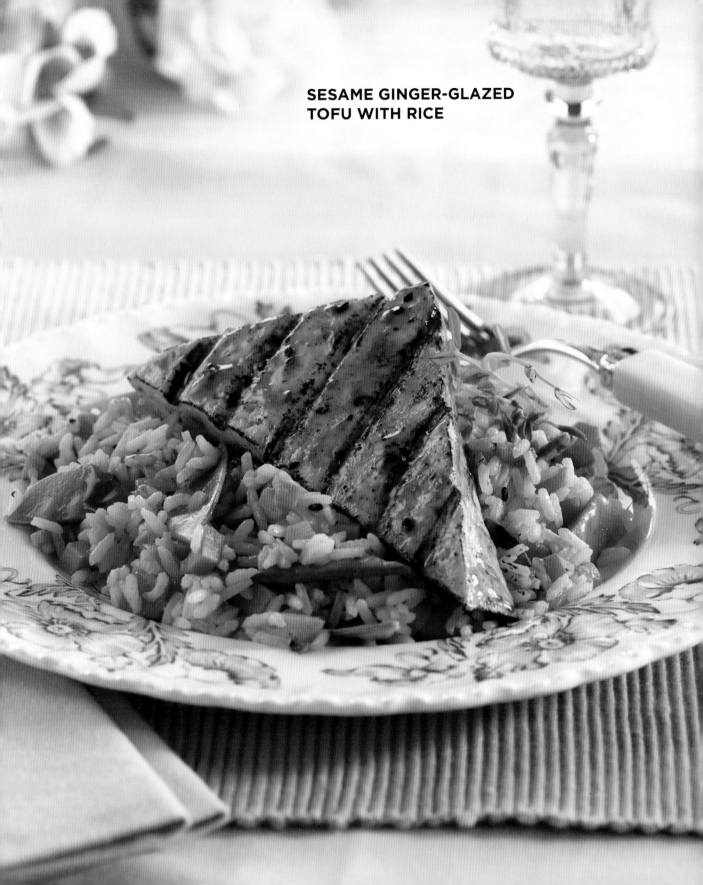

**SESAME GINGER-GLAZED
TOFU WITH RICE**

Mongolian Vegetables

  1 package (about 14 ounces) firm tofu
  4 tablespoons soy sauce, divided
  1 tablespoon dark sesame oil
  1 large head bok choy (about 1½ pounds)
  2 teaspoons cornstarch
  1 tablespoon peanut or vegetable oil
  1 red or yellow bell pepper, cut into short, thin strips
  2 cloves garlic, minced
  4 green onions, cut into ½-inch pieces
  2 teaspoons sesame seeds, toasted*

To toast sesame seeds, spread seeds in small skillet. Shake skillet over medium-low heat 3 minutes or until seeds begin to pop and turn golden.

1. Press tofu lightly between paper towels to drain excess water; cut into ¾-inch squares. Place in shallow dish. Combine 2 tablespoons soy sauce and sesame oil in small bowl; drizzle over tofu. Let stand while preparing vegetables.

2. Cut stems from bok choy leaves; cut stems into ½-inch pieces. Cut leaves crosswise into ½-inch slices.

3. Blend remaining 2 tablespoons soy sauce into cornstarch in small bowl until smooth.

4. Heat peanut oil in wok or large skillet over medium-high heat. Add bok choy stems, bell pepper and garlic; stir-fry 5 minutes. Add bok choy leaves and green onions; stir-fry 2 minutes.

5. Stir cornstarch mixture; add to wok with tofu mixture. Stir-fry 30 seconds or until sauce boils and thickens. Sprinkle with sesame seeds.

Makes 4 servings

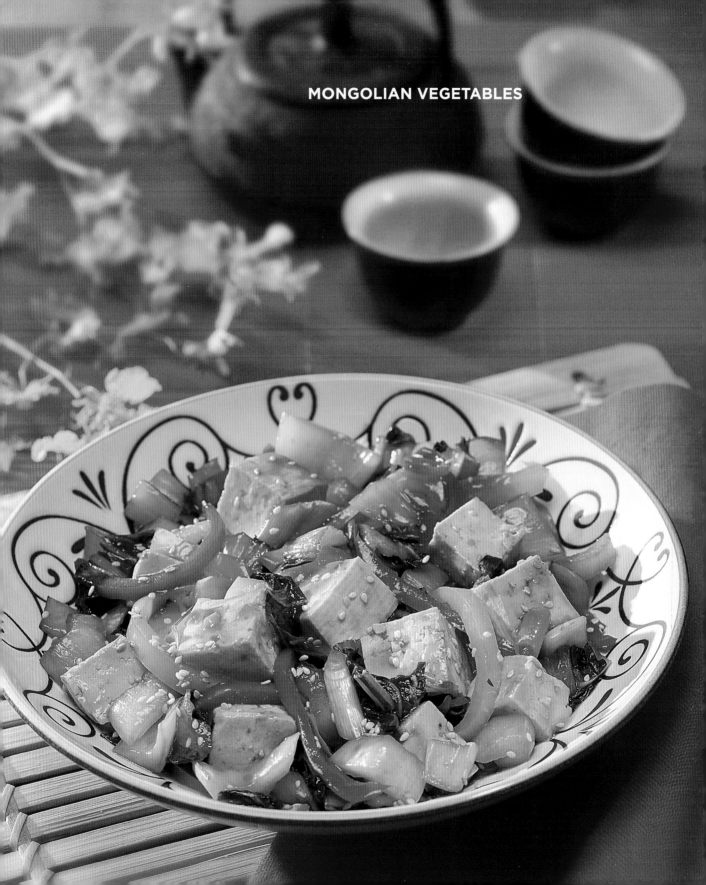
MONGOLIAN VEGETABLES

Tempeh Melt

1 cup water

1 tablespoon hamburger seasoning

1 teaspoon paprika

1 package (8 ounces) unseasoned soy tempeh

Thousand Island Sauce (recipe follows)

4 slices pumpernickel or marble rye bread

Caramelized red onions or red onion slices

Sauerkraut or dill pickle slices

4 slices Swiss cheese

1. Combine water, hamburger seasoning and paprika in large deep skillet. Cut tempeh in half crosswise; add to skillet and bring to a boil over high heat. Reduce heat to low; simmer 20 minutes, turning tempeh occasionally. Remove tempeh from skillet; cut each piece in half.

2. Prepare grill for direct cooking over medium-high heat. Prepare Thousand Island Sauce.

3. Grill tempeh, covered, 4 minutes per side. Spread 1 tablespoon sauce over each of four slices of bread; top with tempeh, caramelized onions and sauerkraut. Top with cheese; if desired, grill sandwiches 30 seconds or until cheese melts.

Makes 4 servings

Thousand Island Sauce: Combine ½ cup mayonnaise, ½ cup chili sauce, 1 tablespoon sweet pickle relish, 2 teaspoons Dijon mustard and dash ground red pepper in food processor; process until smooth.

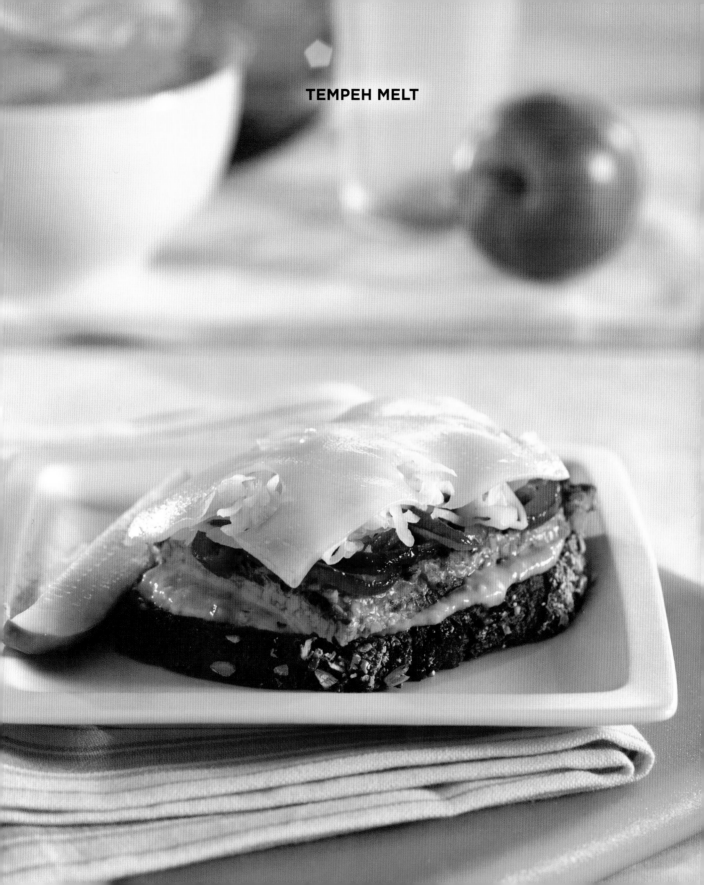

TEMPEH MELT

Asian Noodle Skillet

    4 ounces soba (buckwheat) noodles
    2 tablespoons vegetable oil, divided
    1 pound firm tofu, cut into 1-inch cubes
    4 cloves garlic, minced
    1 tablespoon minced fresh ginger
    1 can (8 ounces) water chestnuts
    1 cup baby corn
 1½ cups mushroom or vegetable broth
    2 tablespoons soy sauce
    1 cup snow peas
  ¼ cup green onions, thinly sliced

1. Bring about 6 cups water to boil in large saucepan over high heat. Add noodles; boil 1 minute or until wilted, stirring to separate noodles. Rinse under cold water and drain.

2. Heat 1 tablespoon oil in large nonstick skillet over medium-high heat. Add tofu; cook until browned on all sides. Remove to plate. Add remaining 1 tablespoon oil to skillet. Add garlic and ginger; cook and stir about 1 minute or until fragrant. Stir in water chestnuts and corn.

3. Return browned tofu to skillet. Add broth, soy sauce, snow peas and noodles; bring to a boil. Reduce heat to medium-low; simmer 3 minutes or until noodles are cooked through and most of liquid has evaporated. Stir in green onions.

Makes 4 servings

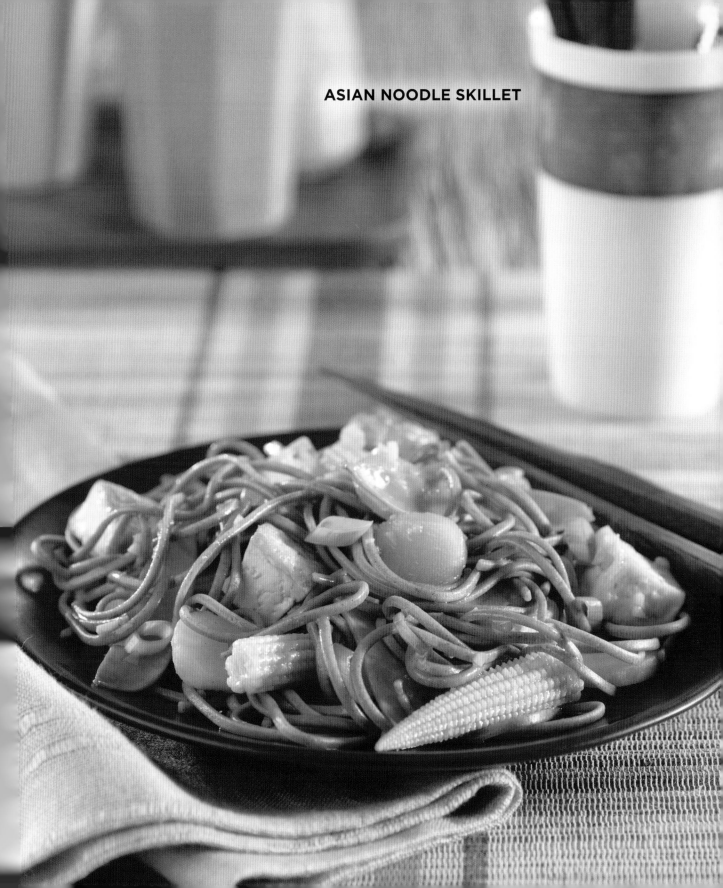

ASIAN NOODLE SKILLET

Ma Po Tofu

1 package (14 ounces) firm tofu, drained and pressed*

2 tablespoons soy sauce

2 teaspoons minced fresh ginger

1 cup vegetable broth, divided

2 tablespoons black bean sauce

1 tablespoon Thai sweet chili sauce

1 tablespoon cornstarch

2 tablespoons vegetable oil

1 green bell pepper, cut into bite-size pieces

2 cloves garlic, minced

1½ cups broccoli florets

¼ cup chopped fresh cilantro (optional)

Hot cooked rice

*Cut tofu in half horizontally and place between layers of paper towels. Place a weighted cutting board on top; let stand 15 to 30 minutes.

1. Cut tofu into cubes. Place in shallow dish; sprinkle with soy sauce and ginger.

2. Whisk ¼ cup broth, black bean sauce, chili sauce and cornstarch in small bowl until smooth and well blended; set aside.

3. Heat oil in wok or large skillet over high heat. Add bell pepper and garlic; stir-fry 2 minutes. Add remaining ¾ cup broth and broccoli; bring to a boil. Reduce heat to medium-low; cover and simmer 3 minutes or until broccoli is crisp-tender.

4. Stir sauce mixture; add to wok. Cook 1 minute or until sauce boils and thickens. Stir in tofu; cook until heated through. Sprinkle with cilantro, if desired. Serve with rice.

Makes 4 servings

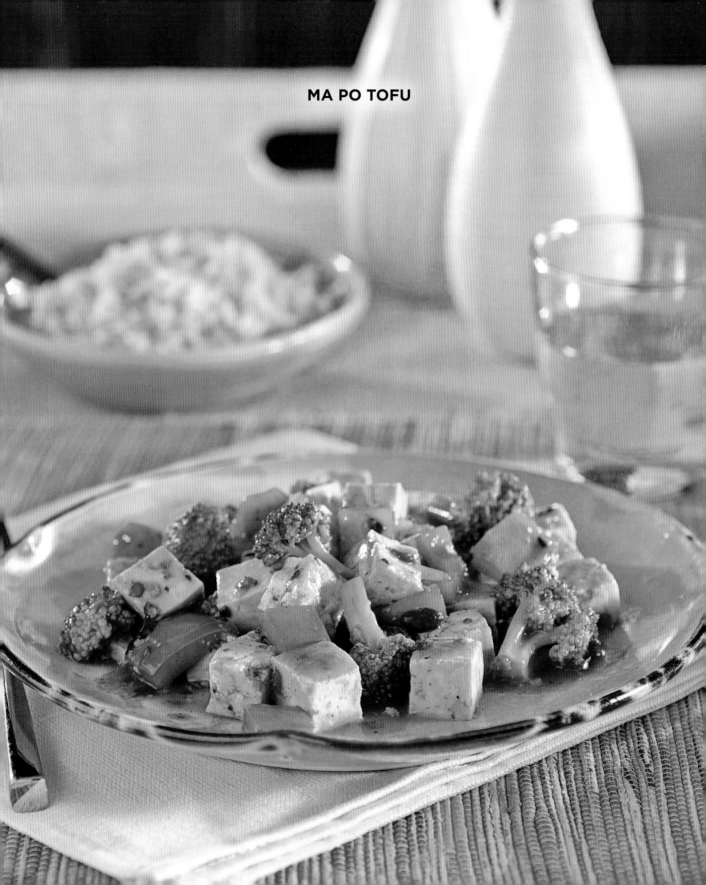

MA PO TOFU

Seitan Fajitas

1 package (1 ounce) fajita seasoning mix

2 packages (8 ounces each) seitan,* sliced

1 tablespoon vegetable oil

1 red bell pepper, sliced

½ medium onion, sliced

1 package (8 ounces) sliced mushrooms

6 (6- to 7-inch) tortillas, warmed

Salsa and sour cream (optional)

1. Dissolve fajita seasoning according to package directions. Place seitan in large resealable food storage bag; pour seasoning mixture over seitan. Seal bag; shake to coat.

2. Heat oil in large skillet over medium-high heat. Add bell pepper and onion; cook and stir 4 to 5 minutes or until crisp-tender. Add mushrooms; cook and stir 3 minutes or until mushrooms are softened. Add seitan and seasoning mixture; cook and stir 1 to 2 minutes or until seitan is heated through and vegetables are coated with seasoning.

3. Divide vegetable mixture evenly among tortillas. Serve with salsa and sour cream, if desired.

Makes 6 fajitas

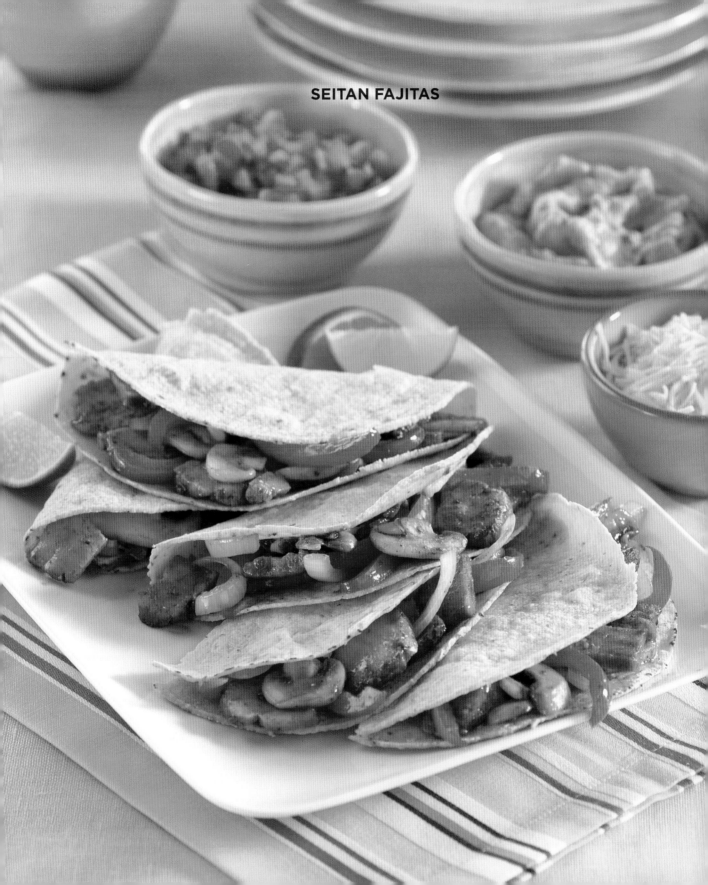

SEITAN FAJITAS

Tofu Stuffed Shells

- 1 can (15 ounces) tomato purée
- 8 ounces mushrooms, thinly sliced
- ½ cup shredded carrot
- ¼ cup water
- 2 cloves garlic, minced
- 1 tablespoon sugar
- 1 tablespoon Italian seasoning
- 12 uncooked jumbo pasta shells
- 1 package (14 ounces) firm tofu, drained and pressed
- ½ cup chopped green onions
- 2 tablespoons grated Parmesan cheese
- 2 tablespoons minced fresh parsley
- 1 tablespoon dried basil
- ½ teaspoon salt
- ¼ teaspoon black pepper
- ½ cup (2 ounces) shredded mozzarella cheese

1. Combine tomato purée, mushrooms, carrot, water, garlic, sugar and Italian seasoning in medium saucepan; bring to a boil over medium-high heat. Reduce heat to low; cover and simmer 20 minutes, stirring occasionally.

2. Meanwhile, cook shells according to package directions; drain. Preheat oven to 350°F. Spread thin layer of sauce in bottom of 11×8-inch baking pan.

3. Crumble tofu into medium bowl. Stir in green onions, Parmesan, parsley, basil, salt and pepper; mix well. Stuff shells with tofu mixture (about 1 heaping tablespoon per shell). Place shells, stuffed side up, in single layer in prepared pan. Pour remaining sauce over shells. Cover pan tightly with foil.

4. Bake 30 minutes. Remove foil; sprinkle with mozzarella. Bake, uncovered, 5 to 10 minutes or until hot and bubbly.

Makes 4 servings

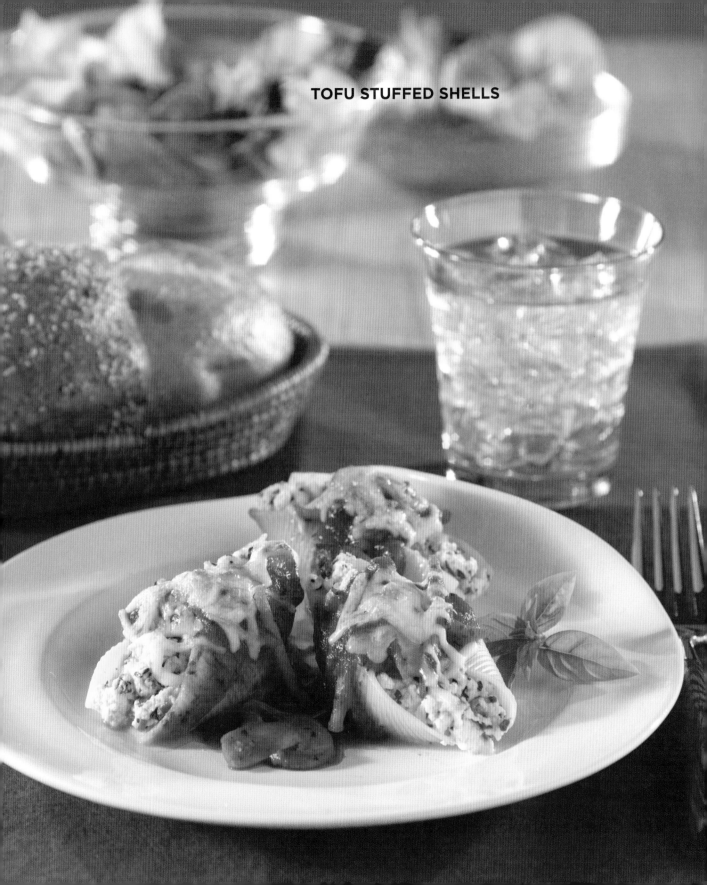
TOFU STUFFED SHELLS

Tofu and Snow Pea Noodle Bowl

  5 cups water

  6 tablespoons chicken-flavored broth powder*

  4 ounces uncooked vermicelli, broken in thirds

  8 ounces firm tofu, rinsed, drained and cut into ¼-inch cubes

  1 cup (3 ounces) fresh snow peas

  1 cup matchstick-size carrot strips**

  ½ teaspoon Chinese chili-garlic sauce

  ½ cup chopped green onions

  ¼ cup chopped fresh cilantro (optional)

  2 tablespoons lime juice

  1 tablespoon grated fresh ginger

  2 teaspoons soy sauce

Chicken-flavored vegetarian broth powder can be found in natural food stores and some supermarkets.

**Matchstick-size carrot strips are sometimes called shredded carrots and may be sold with other prepared vegetables in the supermarket produce section.

1. Bring water to a boil in large saucepan over high heat. Stir in broth powder and vermicelli; return to a boil. Reduce heat to medium; cook 6 minutes. Stir in tofu, snow peas, carrots and chili-garlic sauce; cook 2 minutes.

2. Remove from heat; stir in green onions, cilantro, if desired, lime juice, ginger and soy sauce. Serve immediately.

Makes 4 servings

Tip: Substitute 5 cups of canned vegetarian chicken-flavored broth for the water and broth powder.

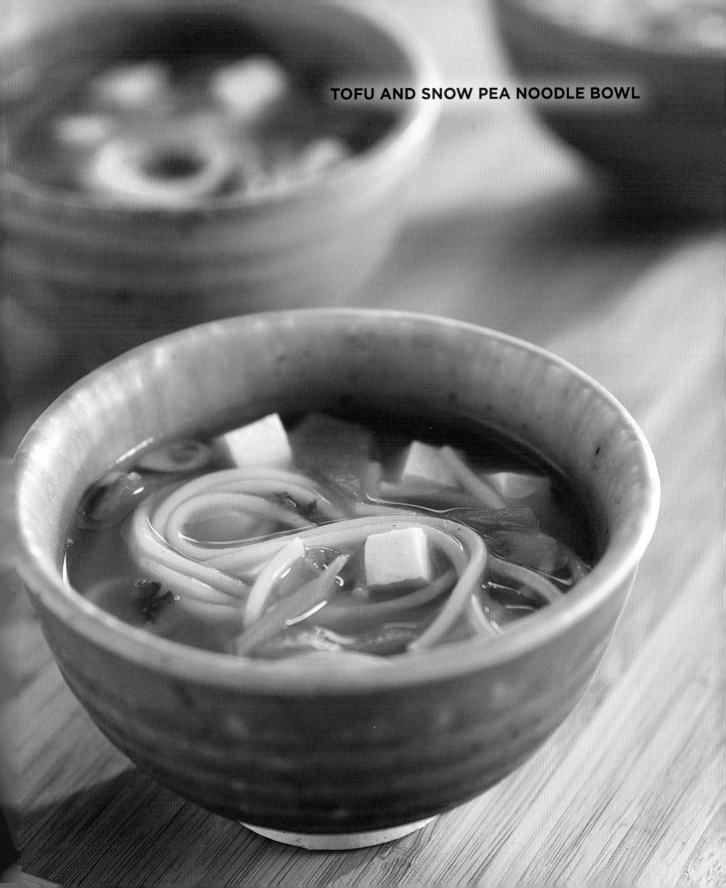

TOFU AND SNOW PEA NOODLE BOWL

Thai Seitan Stir-Fry

  1 package (8 ounces) seitan, drained and thinly sliced
  1 jalapeño pepper, halved and seeded
  3 cloves garlic
  1 piece peeled fresh ginger (about 1 inch)
  ⅓ cup soy sauce
  ¼ cup packed brown sugar
  ¼ cup lime juice
  ½ teaspoon red pepper flakes
  ¼ teaspoon salt
  3 tablespoons vegetable oil
  1 medium onion, chopped (about 2 cups)
  2 red bell peppers, quartered and thinly sliced (about 2 cups)
  2 cups fresh broccoli florets
  3 green onions, diagonally sliced
  4 cups lightly packed baby spinach
  ¼ cup shredded fresh basil
  3 cups hot cooked rice
  ¼ cup salted peanuts, chopped

1. Place seitan in medium bowl. Combine jalapeño, garlic and ginger in food processor; process until finely chopped. Add soy sauce, brown sugar, lime juice, red pepper flakes and salt; process until blended. Pour mixture over seitan; stir to coat. Marinate at room temperature at least 20 minutes.

2. Heat oil in wok or large skillet over high heat. Add chopped onion, bell peppers and broccoli; stir-fry 3 to 5 minutes. Add seitan with marinade and green onions; bring to a boil. Cook and stir 3 minutes or until vegetables are crisp-tender and seitan is heated through. Add half of spinach; cook just until beginning to wilt. Add remaining spinach; cook just until wilted.

3. Stir in basil just before serving. Serve over rice; sprinkle with peanuts.

Makes 4 to 6 servings

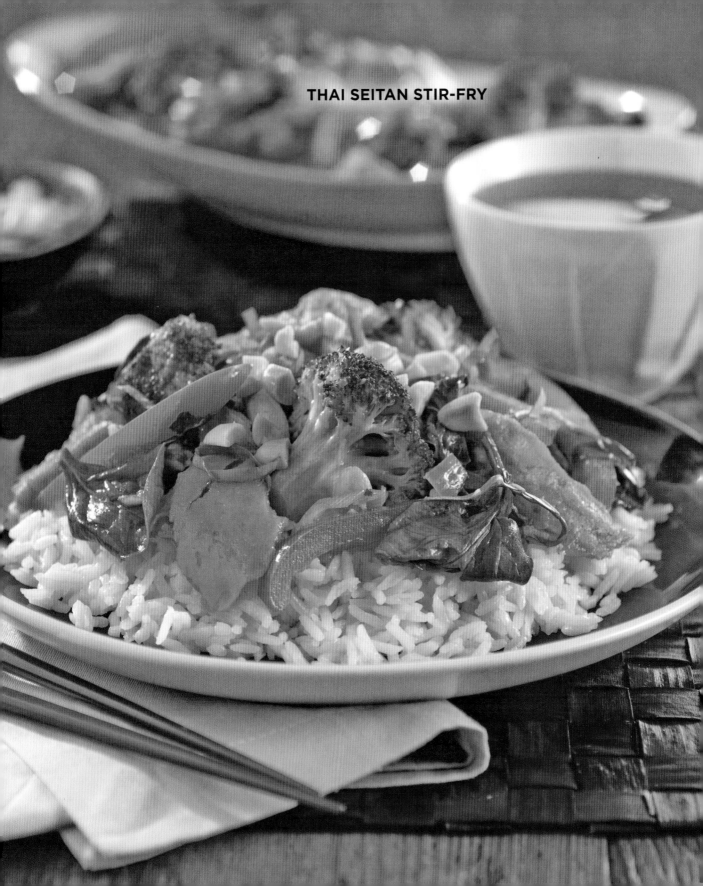

THAI SEITAN STIR-FRY

Spaghetti with Pesto Tofu Squares

1 package (14 ounces) extra firm tofu

¼ to ½ cup prepared pesto

½ (16-ounce) package uncooked spaghetti

1 jar (24 ounces) marinara sauce

½ cup shredded Parmesan cheese

¼ cup pine nuts, toasted*

*To toast pine nuts, spread in shallow baking pan. Bake in preheated 350°F oven 5 to 7 minutes or until golden brown, stirring frequently. Immediately remove from pan; cool before using.

1. Preheat oven to 350°F. Spray shallow baking dish with nonstick cooking spray.

2. Cut tofu into 1-inch cubes. Combine tofu and pesto in medium bowl; toss to coat. Spread in prepared baking dish. Bake 15 minutes.

3. Meanwhile, cook spaghetti according to package directions; drain and return to saucepan. Add marinara sauce; toss to coat. Cover and cook 5 minutes over low heat or until heated through.

4. Divide spaghetti among four plates; top with tofu cubes. Sprinkle with cheese and pine nuts.

Makes 4 servings

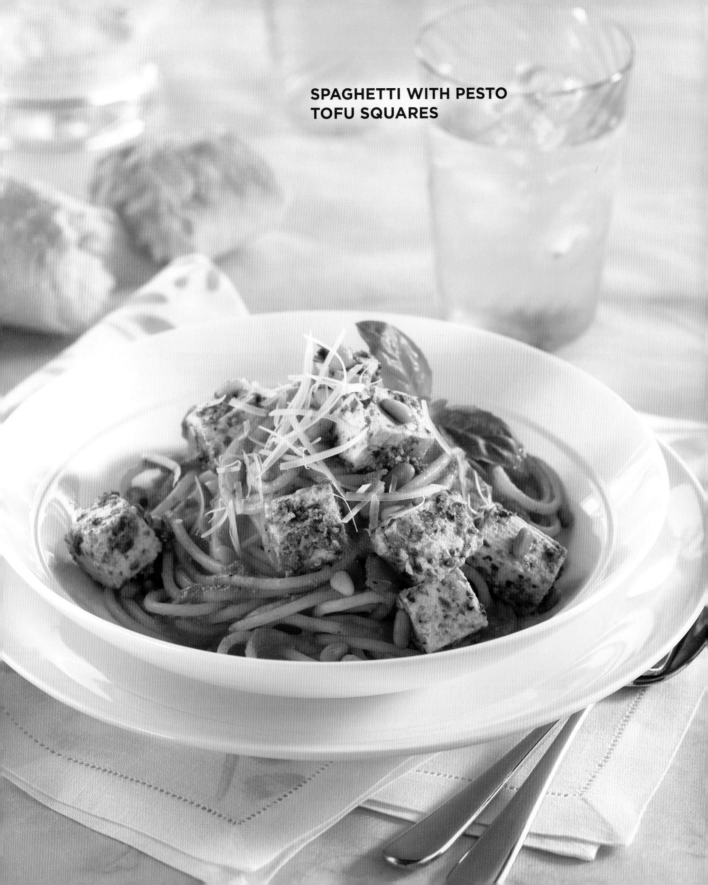

SPAGHETTI WITH PESTO TOFU SQUARES

Summer Szechuan Tofu Salad

¼ cup reduced-sodium soy sauce

1 tablespoon canola or peanut oil

1 tablespoon dark sesame oil

1 teaspoon minced fresh ginger

½ teaspoon hot pepper sauce or more to taste

1 package (14 ounces) extra firm tofu

4 cups baby spinach leaves

4 cups sliced napa cabbage or romaine lettuce

2 cups fresh snow peas or sugar snap peas, cut into halves

1 cup matchstick-size carrots

1 cup fresh bean sprouts

¼ cup dry-roasted peanuts or toasted slivered almonds

Chopped fresh cilantro or green onions (optional)

1. Combine soy sauce, canola oil, sesame oil, ginger and hot pepper sauce in small bowl; mix well.

2. Drain tofu and place between two paper towels; press lightly to drain excess water. Cut tofu into 1-inch cubes; place in shallow dish. Drizzle with 2 tablespoons soy sauce mixture.

3. Combine spinach, cabbage, snow peas, carrots and bean sprouts in large bowl. Add remaining soy sauce mixture; toss to coat. Top with tofu mixture, peanuts and cilantro, if desired.

Makes 4 servings

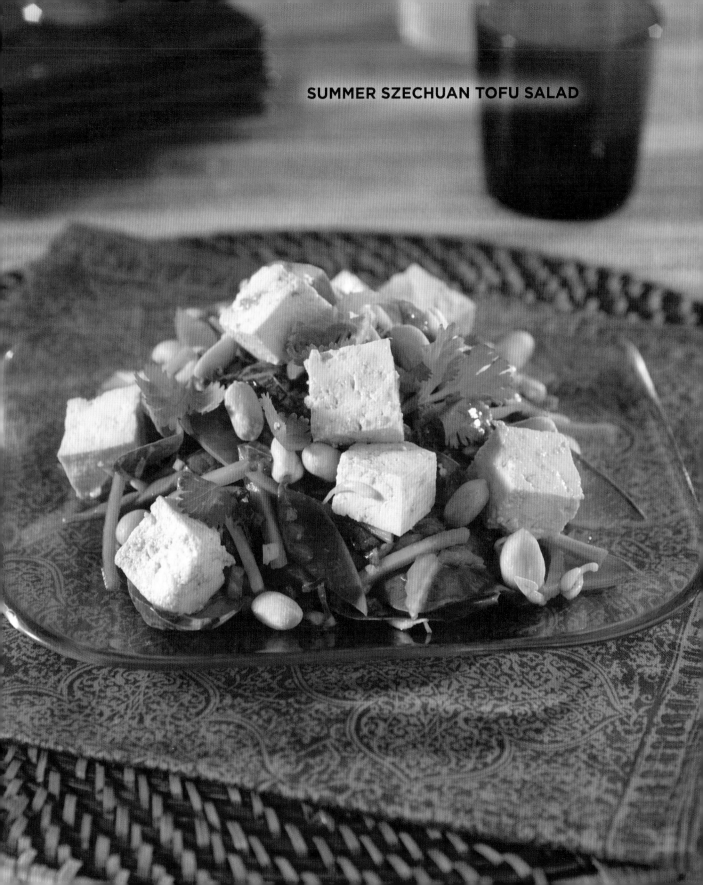

Black Bean and Tempeh Burritos

  2 teaspoons olive oil

  ½ cup chopped onion

  ½ cup chopped green bell pepper

  2 cloves garlic, minced

  2 teaspoons chili powder

  2 cans (about 14 ounces each) stewed tomatoes

  1 teaspoon dried oregano

  ½ teaspoon dried coriander

  1 can (about 15 ounces) black beans, rinsed and drained

  4 ounces tempeh, diced

  ¼ cup minced onion

  ¼ teaspoon black pepper

  ½ teaspoon ground cumin

  8 (6-inch) flour tortillas

1. Heat oil in large nonstick skillet over medium heat. Add chopped onion, bell pepper and garlic; cook and stir 5 minutes or until onion is tender. Add chili powder; cook and stir 1 minute. Add tomatoes, oregano and coriander; cook 15 minutes, stirring frequently.

2. Preheat oven to 350°F. Spray 13×9-inch baking dish with nonstick cooking spray. Place beans in medium bowl; mash well with fork. Stir in tempeh, minced onion, black pepper and cumin. Add ¼ cup sauce; mix well.

3. Soften tortillas, if necessary.* Spread ⅓ cup bean mixture down center of each tortilla. Roll up tortillas; place in single layer in prepared baking dish. Top with remaining sauce.

4. Bake 15 minutes or until heated through.

To soften tortillas, wrap stack of tortillas in foil. Heat in preheated 350°F oven about 10 minutes or until softened.

Makes 4 servings

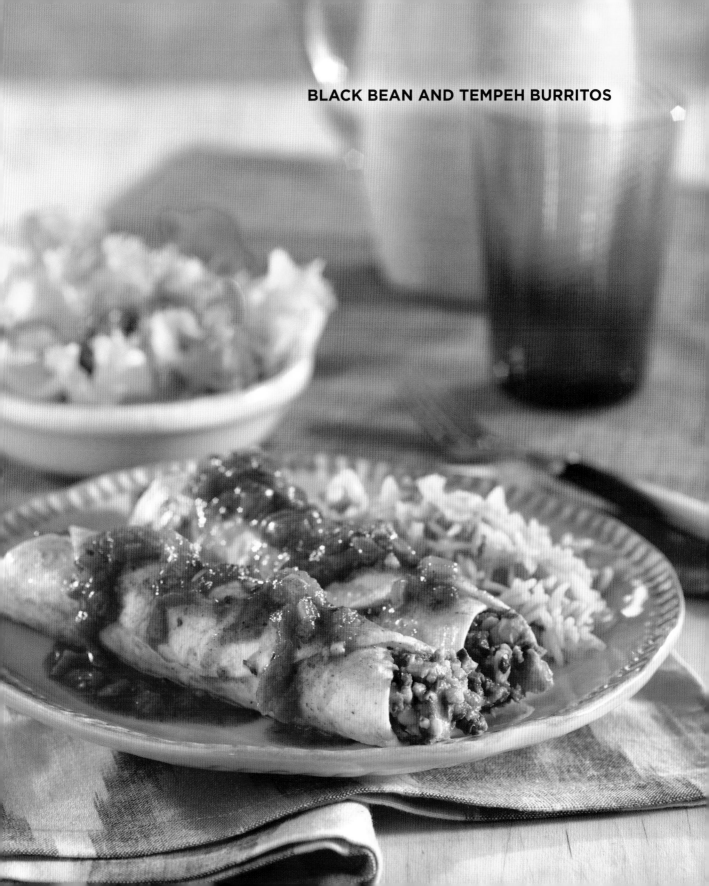

BLACK BEAN AND TEMPEH BURRITOS

Thai Veggie Curry

2 tablespoons vegetable oil

1 onion, quartered and thinly sliced

1 tablespoon Thai red curry paste (or to taste)

1 can (about 13 ounces) unsweetened coconut milk

2 red or yellow bell peppers, cut into strips

1½ cups cauliflower and/or broccoli florets

1 cup fresh snow peas

1 package (about 14 ounces) tofu, pressed* and cut into 1-inch cubes

Salt and black pepper

¼ cup slivered fresh basil

Hot cooked jasmine rice

Cut tofu in half horizontally and place between layers of paper towels. Place a weighted cutting board on top; let stand 15 to 30 minutes.

1. Heat oil in large skillet or wok over medium-high heat. Add onion; cook and stir 2 minutes or until softened. Add curry paste; cook and stir to coat onion. Add coconut milk; bring to a boil, stirring to dissolve curry paste.

2. Add bell peppers and cauliflower; cook over medium heat 4 to 5 minutes or until crisp-tender. Stir in snow peas; cook 2 minutes. Gently stir in tofu; cook until heated through.

3. Sprinkle with basil; serve with rice.

Makes 4 to 6 servings

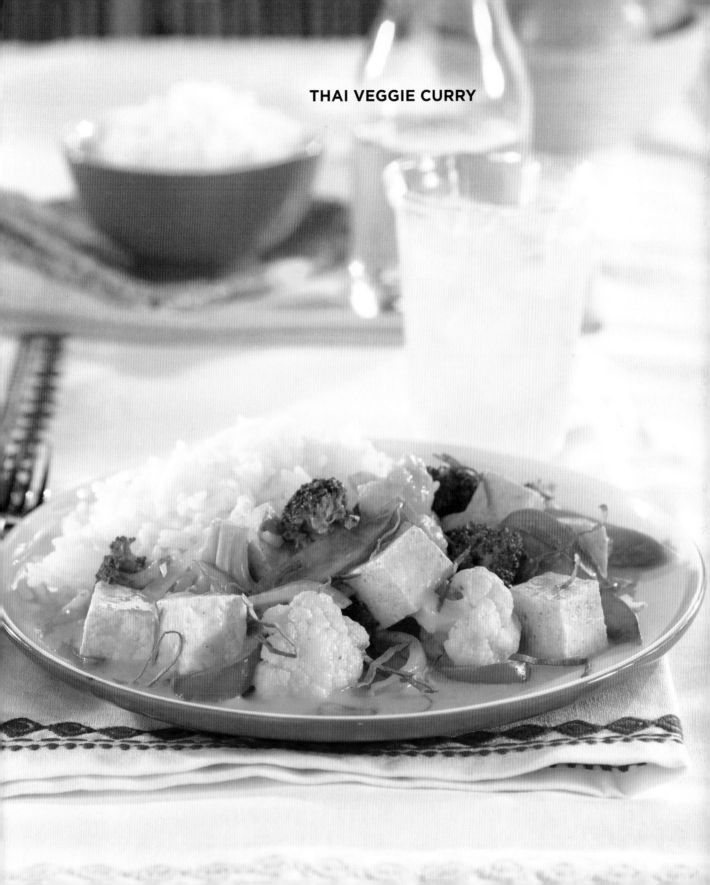

THAI VEGGIE CURRY

Tofu Satay with Peanut Sauce

Satay

  1 package (14 ounces) firm tofu, drained and pressed*

  ⅓ cup water

  ⅓ cup soy sauce

  1 tablespoon sesame oil

  1 teaspoon minced garlic

  1 teaspoon minced fresh ginger

24 white mushrooms, trimmed

  1 large red bell pepper, cut into 12 pieces

Peanut Sauce

  1 can (14 ounces) unsweetened coconut milk

  ½ cup creamy peanut butter

  2 tablespoons packed brown sugar

  1 tablespoon rice vinegar

  1 to 2 teaspoons red Thai curry paste

Cut tofu in half horizontally and place between layers of paper towels. Place a weighted cutting board on top; let stand 15 to 30 minutes.

1. Cut tofu into 24 cubes. Combine water, soy sauce, sesame oil, garlic and ginger in small bowl; mix well. Place tofu, mushrooms and bell pepper in large resealable food storage bag. Add soy sauce mixture; seal bag and turn gently to coat. Marinate 30 minutes, turning occasionally. Soak eight 8-inch bamboo skewers in water 20 minutes.

2. Preheat oven to 400°F. Spray 13×9-inch glass baking dish with nonstick cooking spray.

3. Drain tofu mixture; discard marinade. Thread skewers, alternating tofu with mushrooms and bell pepper. Place skewers in prepared baking dish.

4. Bake 25 minutes or until tofu is lightly browned and vegetables are tender.

5. Meanwhile, combine coconut milk, peanut butter, brown sugar, vinegar and curry paste in small saucepan; bring to a boil over medium heat, stirring constantly. Reduce heat to low; cook about 20 minutes or until creamy and thick, stirring frequently. Serve skewers with sauce.

Makes 4 servings

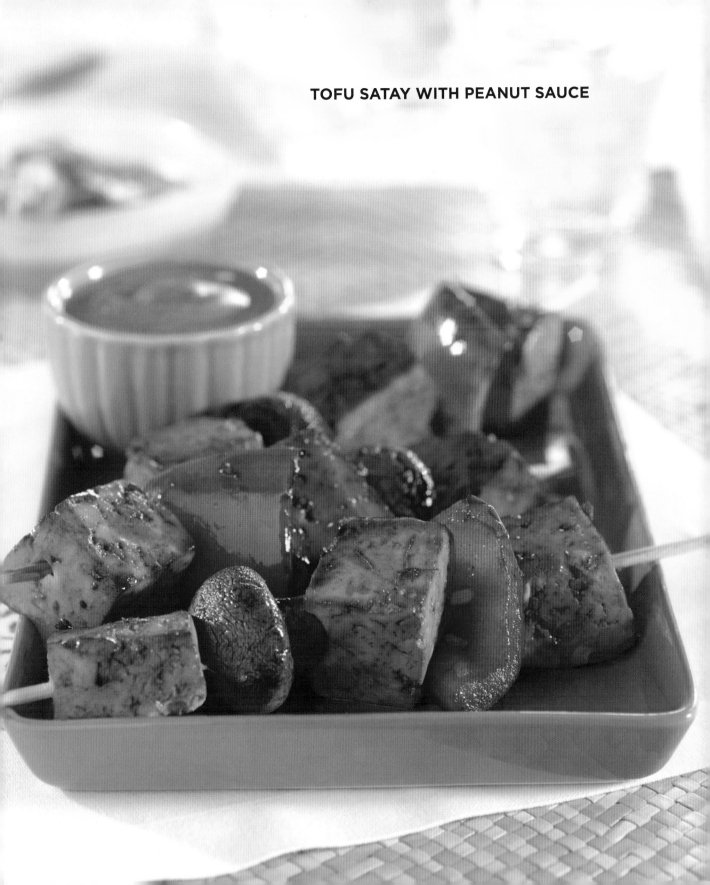

TOFU SATAY WITH PEANUT SAUCE

Index

Index

Index

Index

Index

METRIC CONVERSION CHART

VOLUME MEASUREMENTS (dry)

1/8 teaspoon = 0.5 mL
1/4 teaspoon = 1 mL
1/2 teaspoon = 2 mL
3/4 teaspoon = 4 mL
1 teaspoon = 5 mL
1 tablespoon = 15 mL
2 tablespoons = 30 mL
1/4 cup = 60 mL
1/3 cup = 75 mL
1/2 cup = 125 mL
2/3 cup = 150 mL
3/4 cup = 175 mL
1 cup = 250 mL
2 cups = 1 pint = 500 mL
3 cups = 750 mL
4 cups = 1 quart = 1 L

VOLUME MEASUREMENTS (fluid)

1 fluid ounce (2 tablespoons) = 30 mL
4 fluid ounces (1/2 cup) = 125 mL
8 fluid ounces (1 cup) = 250 mL
12 fluid ounces (1 1/2 cups) = 375 mL
16 fluid ounces (2 cups) = 500 mL

WEIGHTS (mass)

1/2 ounce = 15 g
1 ounce = 30 g
3 ounces = 90 g
4 ounces = 120 g
8 ounces = 225 g
10 ounces = 285 g
12 ounces = 360 g
16 ounces = 1 pound = 450 g

DIMENSIONS

1/16 inch = 2 mm
1/8 inch = 3 mm
1/4 inch = 6 mm
1/2 inch = 1.5 cm
3/4 inch = 2 cm
1 inch = 2.5 cm

OVEN TEMPERATURES

250°F = 120°C
275°F = 140°C
300°F = 150°C
325°F = 160°C
350°F = 180°C
375°F = 190°C
400°F = 200°C
425°F = 220°C
450°F = 230°C

BAKING PAN SIZES

Utensil	Size in Inches/Quarts	Metric Volume	Size in Centimeters
Baking or Cake Pan (square or rectangular)	8×8×2	2 L	20×20×5
	9×9×2	2.5 L	23×23×5
	12×8×2	3 L	30×20×5
	13×9×2	3.5 L	33×23×5
Loaf Pan	8×4×3	1.5 L	20×10×7
	9×5×3	2 L	23×13×7
Round Layer Cake Pan	8×1½	1.2 L	20×4
	9×1½	1.5 L	23×4
Pie Plate	8×1¼	750 mL	20×3
	9×1¼	1 L	23×3
Baking Dish or Casserole	1 quart	1 L	—
	1½ quart	1.5 L	—
	2 quart	2 L	—